The Will to Health
Inertia, Change and Choice

Robert Reynolds, Ph.D, N.D.

Hohm Press

Prescott, Arizona

Cover design: Kim Johansen
Layout and design: Tori Bushert

The author and publisher gratefully acknowledge the use of "Damn Thirsty" by Hafiz, from *The Gift*, by Daniel Ladinsky. Copyright © 1999 by Daniel Ladinsky. Reprinted by permission of the author.

Library of Congress Cataloging-in-Publication Data

Reynolds, Robert, 1950
  The will to health : inertia, change and choice / Robert Reynolds.-- 1st ed.
    p. cm.
  Includes bibliographical references and index.
1. Health--Psychological aspects. 2. Sick--Psychology. 3. Health
    behavior. 4. Will. 5. Medicine and psychology. I. Title.
  R726.5.R49 2004
  613--dc22
2004000184

HOHM PRESS
P.O. Box 2501
Prescott, AZ 86302
800-381-2700
www.hohmpress.com

This book was printed in the U.S.A. on acid-free paper using soy ink.

08 07 06 05 04   5 4 3 2 1

First
The fish needs to say,

"Something ain't right about this
Camel ride —

And I'm
Feeling so damn
Thirsty."

— Hafiz

APPRECIATION

Writing a book does many things. For one, it steadily transforms the mind of the author into a vortex that weaves together everything experienced. In my case, this meant subjecting my extended family to thoughts on the nature of change on a daily basis for over two years. Without your patience, this book would not have been completed.

Most days I was pleasantly surprised by this or that fact about medicine or psychology. What I had not anticipated was that I'd learn, first hand, what it means to struggle with inertia. There are always temptations and rationales for not doing the work. Only after we have breathed life into a project and given it repeated CPR, are we free to take it on a recreational holiday, playing with the ideas and trying them out in different domains. With hindsight, I am grateful for inertia since without resistance to change there cannot be creative resolution.

In any concerted effort of the will we discover our true friends. I benefited every day from your loving support, and, when I became distracted, the gentle reminder that the work was impatiently awaiting my attention.

My confidence was bolstered by Dr. Henry Ahlstrom's scrutiny of the early chapters, and by an understanding editor, Regina Sara Ryan. Special appreciation goes to Kathy Stiles, who thoughtfully read the various versions of each chapter, and who now recalls better than I where a particular passage is located in the text. Nothing is so powerful as one who listens.

Finally, there are those individuals who have shared with me the self-reflections that make up the cases of this book. I have learned much from you, especially in those quiet moments together when you recalled the uncommon feeling of being yourself. Forgive me for camouflaging your brilliant uniqueness for the sake of your privacy. No fictionalizing can do justice to your real life acts of heroism.

CONTENTS

FOREWORD

by David Cumes, M.D.

Healing has been a topic of interest in human society across time and cultures. Many healing rituals have required the ill person to be actively involved in the healing process. In *The Will to Health: Inertia, Change, and Choice* Robert Reynolds develops this basic principle of patient as active participant in making changes that lead to health. This capacity for human choice is often lost sight of in the fog of determinism and the hype of commercialism that pervade so much of our modern thinking and experience.

A discussion of healing must include awareness and integration of the many aspects of human existence. This book clearly meets that requirement. Robert Reynolds is not only a doctor of naturopathic medicine but also a research scientist and a psychologist. Naturopathic medicine is a unique, evidence-based school of medicine which incorporates such basic principles as doing no harm, addressing the cause, understanding each person's uniqueness, stimulating and supporting the body-mind complex to heal itself, and using education to empower individuals to make meaningful decisions regarding their own health.

Dr. Reynolds is qualified to speak on a subject that is difficult to understand, i.e., what is it that makes us heal? He writes in a scholarly manner that incorporates knowledge, wisdom, and good old-fashioned common sense. In his writing he makes use of his extensive education and keen intellect to provide sage insights about a difficult subject. It is clear he approaches each patient as a unique human being requiring a creative individual approach. There is no dogma or simplistic formula for healing in these pages.

Robert uses both personal cases and examples of historic figures to illustrate the process of change and healing in which a broad range of healing modalities can be used synergistically to good effect. He eloquently describes how to remove obstructions to healing, including the ghosts from the past and the habituations of the present, in order to come into relationship with our own inner voice. It is the acknowledgement of this inner voice that will help us heal.

The fact that healing is a mystery and will probably always remain so requires that we be humble. An anonymous writer once said, "anyone who isn't confused here does not really understand what is going on." Robert devotes a whole chapter to hubris, showing both its positive and negative aspects. For the individual patient some degree of hubris may be necessary to make life changes. As healers, in contrast, humility is one of the most important qualities we can embrace. A big ego is a liability for a healer. In the end we are channeling healing energy from a universal source whose main ingredient is love. The manner in which a healer relates to hubris is a key ingredient in the channeling of this energy.

There is a difference between a healer and a technician. Our Western allopathic system is replete with excellent technicians. There are far fewer good healers. A technician can claim to be an expert needing little input from the patient. However, Robert emphasizes that the relationship between patient and healer should be one of partnering and of doctor as teacher. This cannot occur with integrity without coming to terms with hubris.

Traditional naturopathic medicine embraces the idea of nature as healer or nature as Big Medicine. As Nobel Laureate in Medicine Charles Huggins said: "Nature hides her secrets with consummate modesty and speaks usually in an unintelligible tongue." This seminal book helps unravel that tongue and increases our understanding of the mystery of healing.

CHAPTER ONE

Inertia, Change and Choice

I nertia is the great principle of the physical world. All objects continue their present behavior until running into something, or until their path is forcibly altered. Fortunately, there is a part of each individual that refuses to be considered an object. In fact, a great deal of energy must be expended to make a living animal behave like an inanimate object. Animals have internal combustion engines, sensors connecting them to the outside world, and an anatomy that allows them to alter their path. As far as I know, humans are the only animals that face the heroic decision to change the course of their lives.

It is an oddity that our ability to change an existing behavior or alter our course in life has been met with a fog of theoretical arguments by those in the behavioral sciences. Psychologists, psychiatrists and philosophers have modeled their models on the physics, biology, or technology of their time. Impressed by the Table of Chemical Elements, nineteenth-century psychologists attempted to reduce all conscious experience to elemental sensations, including what they believed to be our erroneous experience of voluntary action. Other scientists, impressed by experiments on the autonomic nervous system, eliminated consciousness in favor of reflexes. Still others, impressed by clinical pathology, argued that the will to act is an illusion wherein we confuse memory of voices from our past for free will in the moment.

Behavioral psychologists "solved" the problem of motivation by eliminating the mind and substituting for it only those behaviors that are observable, along with associated stimuli. After all, no physicist needs to ask why a billiard ball *chooses* its path. The simplicity of the behavioral model was compelling: an external stimulus affects the organism (represented graphically as a box containing reflexes), eliciting a response.

The following fifty years saw a rise and fall of behaviorism. The model gradually became unruly as it attempted to account for real-world complexity. For example, in the classic case of Pavlovian conditioning, a dog hears a bell while being presented with food, leading eventually to its salivating in response to the "conditioned stimulus" of the bell. Under typical experimental conditions, the dog is strapped down. However, should it be freed at the time of bell ringing, the dog will not lie there and drool, but rather run over to where it anticipates the food to arrive. That is to say that the relationship between stimulus and response appears simple only when the mind is obscured and the ability to choose a response limited.

For the past forty years, cognitive psychology has dominated, along with its computer-inspired model. The reason for this is that the computer is technology capable of human-like problem solving, yet, unlike the mind, fully knowable. We can understand the mind, the reasoning goes, by creating flow-charts necessary for a computer to solve human problems. Similar metaphoric reasoning inspired René Descartes in the seventeenth century. Upon seeing the human-like behavior of mechanical robots, Descartes concluded that we are robots (plus a pineal gland to house the soul!).

Looking at a journal article in cognitive psychology one confronts a series of boxes connected by arrows: a flow chart of information describing how a well-oiled cognitive system solves some problem. The computer can view inputted information, make calculations, and choose the best solution to reach specified goals. The exploration of artificial intelligence systems, in conjunction with high-speed processing, has produced chess playing computers capable of beating the best human chess players. Such systems do not, however, resemble human cognitive processing. Moreover, in the complexity of any real-life situation, there is more than one correct path, and each "player" has the capacity to alter the rules and circumstances of the "game" at will.

All modern psychological theories share the assumption that behavior is determined by forces external to the "executive command center" (to use cognitive or military terminology). Such forces come from what we perceive of our external world, from internal dialogue, or from physiologic reactions. The command center itself can learn and develop, but that too is a function of sensory input or "subroutines." Even theorists contemplating consciousness and spirit (e.g., Ken Wilber's *Integral Psychology*) have little to say about *will*, other than it serving as one of many subroutines. There is no place in these theories for a *will* to change itself.

Thousands of careers in psychology have been dedicated to discovering what intelligence is and where it comes from. The consensus is that about seventy percent of one's intelligence comes from genes, leaving the remaining thirty percent the responsibility of one's environment. Unfortunately, in this paradigm nothing is left over for the individual's ability to shape his or her own intelligence.

Consider the following paragraph on Determinism, taken from a recent textbook chapter teaching psychology students the basic assumptions of science.

> …[B]ehavior is solely influenced by natural causes and does not depend on an individual's choice or "free will." If, instead, we assumed that organisms freely decide their

behavior, then behavior truly would be chaotic, because the only explanation for every behavior would be "because he or she wanted to." ...[W]e assume that you cannot freely choose to exhibit a particular personality or respond in a particular way in a given situation. The laws of behavior force you to have certain attributes and to behave in a certain way in a given situation. Anyone else in that situation will be similarly influenced, because that is how the laws of behavior operate. — G.W. Heiman, *Understanding Research Methods and Statistics*.[1]

Heiman's "basic assumption of science" is actually based on several other unfounded assumptions: (a) free will is not "natural," (b) free will, if it existed, would prevent us from understanding behavior, because (c) will is whimsical, and (d) anyone would react the same given the same set of influences. If psychology students were to accept this grand assumption, their field of scientific inquiry would be restricted to observing only those behaviors where choice had been eliminated, restricted, or hidden from view.

The Influence Paradigm

The influence paradigm runs deep. It is fundamental to both Newtonian and quantum mechanics. It is fundamental to all theories of motivation, be they describing behavior of humans or other animals. The paradigm is fundamental to explanations offered by anthropologists or sociologists, as well as interpretations made by professors of art or literature. Indigenous New Guinea culture was corrupted, we are told, by Margaret Mead's dispensing condoms to the natives. Gustave von Aschenbach's infatuation with a beautiful boy (in *Death in Venice*), we are told by critics, is because the character feels death approaching, and because the author, Thomas Mann, had been influenced by Gustav Mahler.

The influence paradigm is the basis of medicine, be it conventional or complementary. Supposedly, we get sick because of invading germs or because the sugar we eat depresses our immune systems. Alzheimer's disease is supposedly caused either by the APOE gene or damage inflicted on the hippocampus of the brain. In homeopathic medicine, one might have a chronic cough with bloody sputum because the person has inherited a tubercular "miasm" or has acquired a "Phosphorus" constitution that can be made whole by taking dilute amounts of phosphorus.

In the twentieth century, physicists and philosophers told us that the last bastion of free will was that of quantum mechanics. In the answer to a famous quantum conundrum, Schroedinger's Cat, trapped in a box with a vial of poison that might be released at any moment, is both dead and alive until someone looks into its box. The notion of dual states of existence, resolved by the act of observation, appeals to magical thinking in adults. Children do not understand this thought-experiment to be a paradox. I've asked kids, and they want to know how the cat got into the box and why it is sitting there quietly: a real cat would either knock over the poison itself or make so much noise that everyone would know it was alive! The experimentalist will answer that the cat has been restrained and anesthetized. It is telling that for the problem to produce a paradoxical outcome, the ability of the cat to act must be eliminated! And what of the hypothetical observer? If the experiment were conducted repeatedly, the experimenter would learn of his or her own complicity in the cat's demise, and would then face a moral dilemma about whether or not to participate.

By contrast to academic theories, social institutions assume that normal people can make responsible decisions that transcend the influence of their circumstances. In the legal system, for example, it is assumed that we are capable of making an independent choice to commit or not to commit a crime except under extraordinary circumstances. For external forces to excuse a crime, they must be extremely controlling or invasive. In regards to internal forces, we are judged as not responsible for a crime only if defective "wiring" or a chemical lesion (i.e., insanity) prevents us from making a reasoned and informed decision.

Despite our ability to make responsible decisions, we are likely to defer responsibility to someone speaking with the voice of authority. In classic experiments by Stanley Milgram following the Nuremberg trials, an authoritative figure in a white lab coat ordered subjects to torture a stranger (actually someone pretending to be tortured). Under these conditions, ninety percent of people eventually chose to cease compliance. However, no subject in these experiments went beyond noncompliance to taking action on behalf of the "tortured" individual. An unexpected and depressing finding was that if the authority figure asserts that he or she will take "full responsibility for the act," most people *will* carry out the order indefinitely.[2]

A few years ago, I was giving a public lecture on body-mind medicine when I was asked my views on clairvoyance and precognition. I responded that these phenomena could potentially be understood scientifically: to the extent that you can observe the network of interactions in a system, you should be able to predict what will happen next. Unfortunately, this glib answer satisfied my audience by appealing to the influence paradigm. Under social pressure to sound erudite, I sunk to an acceptable explanation rather than thinking creatively. It is clear to me now that when one reflects on his or her history and present circumstances, it is possible, from this higher vantage, to *create* new pathways and redirect old ones.

The Power of Our Choices

If we feel unable to affect the events of our own lives, we risk damage to our health. The most common way anxious depression is acquired involves perceiving events of one's world as determined by a force other than one's own will. If one is swept up into an emotionally intense event or has lived within a setting feeling trapped or helpless, then he or she may need professional help to extricate himself or herself.

In the weeks immediately following the September 11th attacks, we heard, first from the media and then echoed by a depressed public, the refrain "Everything has changed," the tacit message being

"…changed in your world without your say." Television images of the World Trade Center's destruction were emblazoned in our consciousness, shocking us like a bolt of lightening in a cloudless sky. What could be more illustrative of acute stress disorder than the scene of New York City pedestrians passively waiting on the street corner and then moving *en masse* as the "Don't Walk" sign changed? From studies on other tragedies, we may predict that fifty percent of those individuals directly involved will continue to suffer anxious depression associated with posttraumatic stress disorder (PTSD).[3] Those in the Oklahoma City bombing who still suffer were those who had felt trapped and unable to affect the drama being played-out about them. Similarly, case studies of concentration camp victims show that the greatest threat of death comes from entering a profound state of depression precipitated by feeling unable to make meaningful choices.

In order to improve a chronic condition, you must make changes.

As indicated above, inertia is the dominant tendency in nature. It is the rare case when someone who is weakened and confused from their disease chooses to change his or her life for the better. It is an unfortunate truth that even those with the capacity to do so, resist making changes to preempt a developing disease. This flies in the face of a basic principle in healthcare: In order to improve a chronic condition, you must make changes.

How is it that doctors continue to prescribe medications shown to yield ten to twenty percent improvement, while knowing that lifestyle changes will double or triple lifespan from the time of diagnosis? In medical parlance, the reason is lack of compliance. Most patients are more likely to take a pill than alter their diet, exercise, meditate, or create new habits and relationships. In fact, a great deal of effort is expended by patients to maintain the very environment and behavior that is causing their disease!

From the patient's point of view, they have put themselves into the hands of an authority who assures them that they have no meaningful option other than compliance. Texts on clinical hypnosis counsel that it is unnecessary to carry out formal hypnotic induction on patients entering a physician's office: they are already in a hypnotic trance and ready for suggestion. From the moment that an individual contacts a physician for help, the doctor has become a central part of the patient's life story. This makes it essential for physicians to be constantly aware that what they say has consequences.

This book contains a collection of stories drawn from my medical practice with an eye to the choices patients make. Sharing stories with my patients helps them to realize that they are engaged in a healing process, that they can become healthier than ever before, and that such healing ultimately depends upon the changes they make. At the first opportunity, I commend my patients for engaging in a heroic decision.

The hero in medicine has always been the patient. Mythological heroes follow a common pattern of development. They leave their comfortable surroundings, either by circumstances or by choice, to confront *the demon*. Faced with many challenges, the hero discovers his personal weaknesses and lack of wholeness. He encounters numerous teachers giving him the annoying message that he has the inner resources to complete the quest. Alone with fear, self-doubt and physical weakness, the hero questions whether confronting *the demon* is worth the risk of death. The ultimate choice to move forward makes the hero whole.

Such stories had long existed as adult instruction before being organized into fairy tales for children. To see how rich these stories are, you might read Robert Bly's telling of Hans Christian Andersen's *Iron John*.[4] Patients struggling with their own demons find useful parallels between these stories and their own.

Mind-Body Relations

Consider the person with a physiological problem metabolizing sugar: his or her blood glucose will go up precipitously after eating sweets. Such circumstances weaken one's ability to resist acting impulsively, be it binge eating or violent retaliation. Most of the time, people will choose to suppress or sublimate socially reprehensible behavior despite the impulse, or to turn down the Twinkie despite craving it. The heroic effort, one that is both rare and life-changing, involves choosing to change one's impulse or craving.

There are many ways by which the mind can influence one's health. In the late nineteenth century, physicians were impressed by the cases of Sigmund Freud and his associates. In hysteria, patients exhibit debilitating symptoms with no known physical cause. For example, one of Freud's mentors, Jean Martin Charcot, reported the case of a woman in her late twenties who had had no menstrual period since thirteen years of age. She had been shocked by the occurrence of her first period and had plunged herself into a barrel of icy water in an attempt to wash it away. She became ill and remained unconscious for some days. Upon waking, her memory of events was gone, along with future menstrual cycles. In a brilliant act of hubris, Charcot hypnotized the young woman and planted a false recollection: henceforth she believed that she had had a non-hysterical reaction to a normal body function. This psychic intervention immediately led to a regular menstrual cycle.

Beyond hysterical symptoms, we often find signs of a psychosomatic reaction: a psychological event that causes signs of physiological pathology. In a classic experiment, Ikemi and Nakagawa (1962) hypnotized subjects so as to determine if a skin rash could be affected by one's understanding. One group was given the false suggestion that they were touching a toxic wax-tree leaf: under hypnosis, they quickly developed a rash on their hands. Another group was misled into believing that they were handling a chestnut leaf when, in fact, they were touching a wax-tree leaf. These subjects did not develop a rash despite the fact that toxic essential oils penetrated their skin.[5] This is just the first of many examples we will consider in which one's immune system is affected by one's mind.

In the past fifty years or so, many diseases have been found to commonly arise from psychosomatic reactions. Moreover, contemporary research on body-mind medicine allows us to explicate the physiological mechanism connecting an emotional stressor with a disease. As an example, let's consider the formation of stomach or intestinal ulcers. For many years, ulcers were the classic example of stress causing physical harm, namely, high levels of acid that eventually wear away the lining of the digestive track.

Before looking at the physiology and biochemistry of ulcer formation, we should note that contemporary medicine has reverted to the nineteenth century germ theory. The idea is that the bacterium *Helicobacter pylorus* is the cause of ulcers; the cure is a combination of antibiotics to kill the bacteria. Holistic practitioners also subscribe to this theory, though they are likely to use herbal antibiotics or nutrients to kill the bug. In fact, ninety percent of all digestive ulcers are found to have *H. pylori* in the wound, though this should not be taken to mean that it is the cause.

On average, ten new articles on ulcers appear each month in medical journals, which provides us a clear picture of the complex

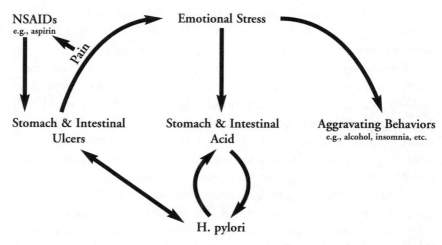

Figure 1.1. Psychosomatic pathways of ulcer formation.

interactions causing ulcers. Figure 1.1 illustrates some of these interactions. Increased levels of stomach and intestinal acid can be caused by tobacco, coffee, alcohol, sugars or missed meals. Emotional stress of all sorts (including lack of sleep) also increases acid levels, while at the same time inhibiting the process by which the body secretes buffering agents to protect the digestive tract. As a secondary problem, stress makes people more likely to consume the acid-producers mentioned above. So, where does *H. pylori* come into play? The bacterium is one factor causing tissue irritation and inflammation. Genetic evidence shows that it has co-evolved with Homo sapiens, serving the function of lowering excessively high acid levels. This is why antibiotic therapies for ulcers inevitably cause gastritis (and prescriptions for antacids). An intensive program of antibiotics eventually yields a period of remission from gastric pain, as antibiotic-resistant strains of *H. pylori* reestablish themselves.

As indicated in Figure 1.1, both excessive acid and *H. pylori* increase stomach and intestinal ulcers. This, in turn, causes pain, leading to even more emotional stress, as well as the desire to use anti-inflammatory medications. We see a number of vicious cycles that perpetuate ulcers. For example, chronic feelings of helplessness in one's job make it more likely to drink coffee or alcohol, which increases stomach acid, *H. pylori*, stomach irritation, inflammation and pain, which, in turn, increases anxious depression. One can help the symptoms by taking anti-anxiety drugs, anti-inflammatories, or antacids, or even by engaging an elaborate program including antibiotics. There are even foods and supplements that help to rebuild eroded digestive tissue. But none of this, in itself, will end the reactive cycle. Ultimately, it boils down to a choice: live with pain, support the companies that will produce the next generation of pharmaceuticals, or create fundamental changes in one's life.

For the most part, vicious cycles are not obviously *vicious* so much as they are course perpetuators existing within a reinforcement loop. For example, infants of every species survive because they have attention-getting skills (e.g., crying, or looking adorable to their caretaker). In general, when the world takes notice and responds to our actions or words, we are likely to repeat that behavior. When the reinforcement (e.g., nursing mom) is in response to one's actions (e.g., crying) rather than an independent time schedule, the behavioral loop (both the crying and the nursing) will increase in frequency. When actions or words are attended to only occasionally (e.g., by an alcoholic parent who might be neglectful) the attention-seeking behavior is almost guaranteed to be repeated indefinitely. Living in such a loop creates an ever-tightening spasm of the social, mental or physiologic organs, one that might eventually manifest as a psychosomatic illness. Often, professional assistance is required in order to realize that one has been living in a Skinner Box, and that there are other choices available.

Medical Paradigms

Throughout history, and in all cultures, there have co-existed contrasting approaches to explaining and treating the sick. Over time, political or ideological change causes an "alternative" medicine to become the standard of conventional practice. From the vantage of the prevailing paradigm, historians will marginalize and eventually footnote out of existence an alternative paradigm. However, at any one moment in time, one can find contrasting medical philosophies practiced by competing physicians and available to the public.

Contemporary analysis of just about any topic will divide the world into two groups. As one historian expressed it, "There are two types of people: those who divide the world into two types, and those who don't!" If we resist this temptation, we can see that in medicine there have always been at least three paradigms: (a) one that emphasizes external forces (e.g., The Germ Theory in Western medicine, Pernicious Influences in Chinese medicine), (b) one that emphasizes internal forces (e.g., the immune system in Western medicine, *Ojas* in Ayurvedic medicine), and (c) one that emphasizes the integration of external and internal forces in ways that may be unique to a given individual (e.g., Hippocrates, Avicenna, Charaka).

Charaka was the earliest of medical practitioners who can be established as a historical figure. Practicing in India, seventh century B.C.E., Charaka systematized Ayurvedic medicine while applying the best of existing external and internal theories. While known as the Father of Medicine, distinctive elements of Charaka's theory exist in the history of Western medicine texts only as a footnote. In some ways we may consider his as well as Avicenna's a fourth medical paradigm: the decisions that patients make and actions they undertake maintain and restore their health in the spiritual, mental and physical domains. It is unfortunate that because a theory places the patient in a position of responsibility and incorporates moral and spiritual discipline, it is considered unfit for scientific enquiry.

An alternative schema for comparing medical paradigms contrasts different approaches that physicians take to treating disease. In the middle half of the twentieth century, *allopathic* medicine became so dominant that it was considered simply to be medicine. *Allopathy* literally means "against the pathologic symptoms," and assumes that the physician's job is to eliminate noxious symptoms, preferably by working against the external or internal forces that underlie them. This is the philosophical position that Hippocrates called the Doctrine of Contraries.

Pharmaceutical reference guides, such as *The Physician's Desk Reference* or *The Physician's General*, organize drugs by their physiologic and biochemical actions. The latter guide lists 107 categories of drug actions starting with the word *anti-*, e.g. anti-biotic, anti-depressant, anti-inflammatory, etc. Zantac, an antacid, was the most prescribed drug before it became approved for over-the-counter sales. Tamoxifen, a popular anti-estrogen, is used to suppress the cancer-promoting effects of estrogen. Premarin is a popular drug used to fight the symptoms associated with menopause by replacing a women's diminished production of estrogen. Iron supplements are prescribed to counteract the feelings of tiredness associated with low levels of iron in the blood. These and thousands of other such allopathic medications act to eliminate undesirable symptoms of disease.

There are several benefits to an allopathic attack on symptoms: (a) it is good in emergency situations where stabilizing and maintaining vitals is critical, (e.g., suppressing the immune system in response to anaphylactic shock), (b) it can provide short-term relief from self-limiting disorders (e.g., relieving a headache), (c) it might be necessary when there is irreversible structural impairment to anatomical or regulatory systems (e.g., supplementing thyroid hormone to those whose thyroid has been irradiated), (d) a large number of patients with the same disease (i.e., diagnostic code) can be prescribed the same medication.

There are disadvantages to the allopathic approach as well. Long-term use of allopathic medications will inhibit the body's natural processes (e.g., by hormone replacement or anti-anxiety drugs). Secondly, debilitating side effects are common. Physicians use broad-spectrum medications in high enough doses to affect everyone within a particular diagnostic category. Since suppression or killing is the goal of the allopathic approach, eventually systems not being targeted are adversely affected. Finally, consider that without symptoms, the cause is out of sight. A basic principle of Oriental medicine that has not survived in the West is that in chronic conditions pain should not be eliminated except as a consequence of

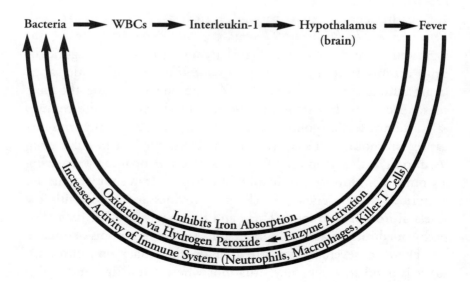

Figure 1.2. Fever as an adaptive response that kills bacteria.

eliminating its cause. By prematurely eliminating unpleasant symptoms, a disease might be maintained at a level acceptable to the physician and patient, thereby precluding a search for the underlying cause.

In contrast to allopathic philosophy, *homeopathy*, along with its stepchild *naturopathy*, view symptoms as the body's attempt to heal itself. As such, the physician's job is to support this process, and, where necessary, stimulate the process of self-healing. *Homeopathy* literally means "similar to the pathologic symptoms," and is the philosophical position that Hippocrates called "Like cures like." From 1800 until the beginnings of World War II, homeopathic and naturopathic medicines were a common alternative to the allopathic approach.

As an example of the appropriateness of homeopathic philosophy, consider how fever is an adaptive response that most often deserves support rather than suppression. An influx of bacteria or viruses will stimulate cells in the brain dedicated to eliciting fever. Figure 1.2 represents a number of pathways by which fever serves to fight a bacterial infection. In fact, most bacteria die off when body temperature rises three or more degrees above normal. At approximately 102 degrees Fahrenheit, enzymes are activated that generate hydrogen peroxide, whose high oxygen content kills invading organisms. Also at that temperature, the immune system becomes maximally mobilized, with increased activity of neutrophils, macrophages, and killer T-cells. At the same time, fever inhibits iron absorption, iron being a favorite fuel for bacteria.

In a recent experiment, volunteers were infected with an influenza virus. Half the group was given medication to reduce fever and other inflammatory symptoms.[6] It should not be surprising that the group treated allopathically experienced flu symptoms for, on average, 3 1/2 days longer than the control subjects who were given no medication. So how should we treat the flu? The naturopathic approach to treating a modest fever entails addressing the cause and gently *raising* the patient's temperature, for example by warm tea, a hot bath, and ginseng (which is warming and immune system stimulating).

The Normative Paradigm

In the years between World Wars, every scientific discipline felt the social and economic pressure to use normative statistics. Only those areas of psychology or medicine that could do so were considered "scientific" and therefore worthy of government support. Where disciplines refused to analyze a patient as a member of a statistical group, their funds were withdrawn. This was a major factor leading to the abandonment of homeopathic and naturopathic colleges.

So ingrained today is the paradigm of normative statistics, that it is assumed that scientific answers must be expressed in terms of a statistical mean, with each individual merely one data point contributing to annoying variability. With the development of normative blood values and the technology to access the inner recesses of the patient's body, "scientific" medicine no longer needed to rely on the subjective report of individuals.

Good medical practice looks at, listens to, and treats individuals.

With the coming of World War II, normative medicine came to dominate, while options within primary care medicine narrowed even further. Medical students completing their course work no longer had the choice of performing internships and residencies at a community clinic. Rather, new graduates earned hours toward their licensure either in a MASH unit, in the emergency room, or by focusing attention on one of a growing number of sub-specialties. War medicine requires expertise in emergency triage, antibiotics that work regardless of patient or bacteria, and vaccinations to prevent disease on a massive scale. Carrying these assumptions into peacetime, physicians were respected by their peers for their ability to rapidly and objectively diagnose a complex case (meaning to correctly identify a patient's diagnostic category), and to typically do so independently of the patient's level of consciousness or intentions.

It is ironic that the shift in paradigm to normative patient evaluation and therapy runs counter to what physicians of *all* philosophies agree: good medical practice looks at, listens to, and treats individuals. This is expressed in the basic homeopathic principle, "Treat the patient, not the disease." At the beginning of the twenty-first century it is apparent that integrating general scientific knowledge with unique factors of the individual patient *is* the science and art of medical practice.

Stories of Change

In the following chapters I have attempted to convey the complex stories of individuals struggling with chronic illness. Chapters 2 through 7 correspond to themes I often see in my practice as a naturopathic physician. Entering into a patient's story is a privileged position to witness the sometimes meandering, sometimes raging flow of life. Every life has many streams that connect the events of the past, present and future. Each stream acts as a theme, providing meaning and a vortex for drawing certain events together in memory. To change course in life means to alter one or more of those streams: engineering a new direction, clearing out dead wood to speed things along, or building a dam as part of a reservoir. Alternatively, you might select, perhaps after years of prevarication, one of many existing streams to carry you who-knows-where.

Each chapter describes a type of investment of attention and energy that diverts from what is needed to make a fundamental change. Some individuals recognize that they have a problem, but believe that they can't make changes (Chapter 2, *I Can't Stop...*). Some individuals have a chronic illness that can be traced to a specific event (e.g., a virus) that affected the body or mind so as to impose either a physical handicap or a narrowing of the individual's perceived options (Chapter 3, *Never Well Since...*). At times, a person, thing or event from the past is "enshrined" by the act of selective attention in such a way as to create physical or mental limitations

(Chapter 4, *Relics and Fossils*).

Doctors witnessing the flow of a patient's life story often can see or hear or feel what the patient cannot. Without being aware of it, a patient's beliefs might be the echo of the voice of a significant person from the past. Sometimes, in the process of therapy, medical as well as psychiatric, the patient reacts toward the therapist as though the latter is a significant player from the past (i.e., "transference"). Recognition of unconscious responses, as they are happening, is critical to successfully freeing patients from their past (Chapter 5, *Ghosts*). An unconscious assumption that dominates many individuals' lives is that, "Anything worth doing must be done perfectly." Often acquired early in life, from one or more "ghosts," this assumption may preclude undertaking anything where a less than perfect outcome is guaranteed (Chapter 6, *Perfection*).

A fundamental block to engaging a healing course is not realizing that one has choices. The narrowing of our vision is sometimes due to the false assumption that we already know what is needed, or that we just need more of what we have (Chapter 7, *Hubris*). Working through an illness has the potential to be a humbling experience for doctor and patient alike. A sure sign that one is on a healing journey is that we learn things we had never anticipated.

The medical cases that are discussed in the following pages are of real people seriously engaged in the process of self-discovery. In some instances it has been several years since I last spoke with them, and I pray that they are doing well. In all cases, I have changed their names so as to protect their ability to freely choose who they will become.

CHAPTER TWO

I Can't Stop...

Knowing that you have a problem, or even having insight into the various factors responsible for it, is very far from a solution. After thirty years of practice, Sigmund Freud came to the realization that gaining insight into the dynamics of one's condition was not helpful unless you are motivated to "work through" that insight. Relatively few of his patients were willing to apply their insights so as to alter the course of their lives. As Freud aged, he realized more and more the extent to which patients work to *maintain* their illness in spite of understanding its pathologic nature. This was profoundly depressing for a man proud of his own genius and the founder of a psychological school holding as a basic tenet that health follows from making unconscious motivations conscious.

Freud allopathically accommodated his depression with stimulant drugs while accommodating apparent holes in his theory of psychoanalysis by creating new theory. For example, his book *Beyond the Pleasure Principle* argues that, beyond a drive to achieve a pleasurable release of tension, the most all-encompassing instinct directs us toward death and dissolution. It certainly did not bring Freud pleasure that his students and colleagues rejected his call for a new theory. His critics argued that he had been *influenced* to invoke a death instinct by seeing his sons march off to World War I.

For all of his theoretical accommodations, Freud refused to alter course in his various life "streams" even when his life was threatened. Consequently, he witnessed the course of his life taken out of his own hands: expulsion by Nazis from his beloved home in Vienna, an ever-increasing need for stimulants, and the periodic loss of his voice to cancer of the mouth (the soft palate). After thirty-three surgeries and 350,000 cigars, Freud still refused to stop smoking. He attempted to discover his unconscious motives behind the addiction, but eventually resigned himself to the now-famous statement, "Sometimes a cigar is just a cigar."

In response to his physicians' recommendation to stop smoking, his decision was not *I can't stop* so much as it was *I refuse to stop*. His psychoanalytic colleagues actually encouraged his cigar smoking, smuggling the finest Cuban cigars past the embargoes imposed by his family and the Nazi regime. We might question the motives of his colleagues who, after all, had endured Freud's patronizing insistence that everyone in his circle must also smoke cigars. When not speaking with his cronies, Freud offered a less than ethereal explanation for his not stopping: so long as he defied authority, he could show that he was still in command of his body and mind.

"I can't stop," while sometimes accurately reflecting a physical impossibility, more often is obfuscation. It is a shorthand statement with many possible meanings. For Freud, it meant, "I refuse," expressed with disdain for the authority making the recommendation. Alternatively, it might mean, "I won't stop," a prediction of one's future behavior based on past successes (e.g., persevering in a long-term relationship) or failures. As one of my patients reflected,

"I can't stop eating sweets because I've tried many times and always fail." Notice in this statement the mixing of past and present tenses, as well as the verb "to try," which typically implies failure.

"I can't stop" might also mean, "I shouldn't stop" (i.e., I would be breaking the rules if I did), "I dare not stop" (i.e., The consequences of stopping could be frightening), or "Sorry, but I can't slow down long enough to listen." In practice, when speaking to a therapist individuals are likely to express their refusal to stop as a reasoned choice (i.e., "I choose not to stop"). In order to decipher such a statement, it is necessary for the therapist to know how the individual normally expresses himself or herself. One of my patients repeatedly asserted, "After weighing all the options, I know that I could never leave my husband." The third time I heard this statement, I asked about those "options"; this elicited anger and an unusual tirade of personal attacks; she immediately apologized profusely. It was apparent that her "choice" to stay married was a sham that served to protect her from the consequences of breaking the rules or encountering fear of the unknown.

The inability to stop can affect health in a number of ways. It may involve the perpetuation of a risky behavior like smoking. Or, the continuation of certain behaviors may distract one from engaging in or seeing the need for healthy endeavors. Eventually it drains one's energy to such an extent as to preclude the exercise of behaviors that one knows to be health giving. The word *stop* comes from the Latin *stuppare* and the Greek *stuppe* meaning to plug a hole with fibrous material (e.g., from old ropes) so as to seal a leaking boat. Choosing to stop the loss of vital energy is often the first step in regaining health.

Before reviewing the cases that follow, it is important to ask, "What is health?" Freud was asked this question toward the end of his life. With cigar in hand, he answered rasply, "To love and to work." Today, we can expand Freud's observation since we know that men and women are at increased risk of disease when they are frustrated in their work or love relationships. A recent study found that men, on average, have two and one-half times the likelihood of a heart attack when they feel under-appreciated at work. Women, on average, have three times the risk when experiencing stress in their marriage. However, times are changing, and we are finding more men whose health is deteriorating from insufficient love at home, and increasing numbers of women producing disease out of workplace frustration.

The English word *health* is derived from the Anglo Saxon *hal,* meaning whole. Hippocrates argued that the nature of health is *physis* (from which we get the word *physician*), meaning that in a healthy organism the various parts are functioning together and in harmony with its environment. This is consistent with classical homeopathy and Oriental medical systems that generally have taken health to mean a harmonious balance. For example, in Ayurvedic medicine of India and Tibet, all things, including one's self, are comprised of three forces: (a) that which maintains structure (*Kapha*), (b) that which digests things (*Pitta*), and (c) that which moves us (*Vata*). Supposedly, spiritual, mental and physical disease arise when our actions cause one or more of these forces to dominate.

There are at least three types of imbalances that are studied in Western psychosomatic medicine. The most psychological of these is the potential imbalance between *self* and *other*. We are best able to work and to love when nurturing ourselves without being self-possessed or childishly egocentric. This requires psychosocial boundaries that are neither so porous that one loses one's self, nor so insulating that the boundaries cannot be penetrated. As they say in New England, "Good fences make for good neighbors."

A potential imbalance may also exist in the exchange between what goes in and what comes out of us. A healthy system assimilates and metabolizes essential elements from the world, while returning the byproducts of digestion to the environment. At my healthiest, when eating a piece of salmon, for example, I assimilate its amino acids, short-chained fatty acids, and other nutrients, after which I eliminate waste products through the bowels. At the same time, I pray that I can appreciate the care put into the food's preparation, and express that appreciation to the cook.

Besides a potential problem in the digestion of food, imbalances can arise in two other bodily areas in which we exchange with the world. A healthy system is able to breathe in oxygen and blow off carbon dioxide in such a way as to maintain an optimal acid level. Not only is a diseased state apparent in the breath, but breathing exercises are also a powerful tool to restoring health. The other system that is a source of exchange between our body and the external world is skin. Our skin is a semi-permeable membrane that provides some protection to the inner body; it is instrumental to maintaining a stable internal temperature; it is stimulated by sunlight and thereby instrumental to the production of vitamin D; it is essential to the elimination of waste products through sweat.

The third type of potential imbalance occurs within a nervous system governed by a primitive area of the brain stem. The autonomic or "automatic" nervous system is not dependent upon conscious decisions (though it can be affected by them), e.g., digestion, blood pressure, genital arousal, or panic. Actually, there are two, complementary, autonomic nervous systems. The sympathetic nervous system is "sympathetic" to the immediate needs of the organism; it gets us up for what it senses to be a dangerous encounter, for

---

In general, we digest food, store nutrients, engage cellular metabolism (creating energy), and regenerate tissues only to the extent that we are in a parasympathetic mode.

---

example causing dilated pupils, sweaty palms, racing heart, shallow breath, and a hypervigilant mind. When confronted with a stressful situation, the body moves blood away from the heart, brain and digestive organs, and out to the muscles of the arms and legs, thereby increasing blood pressure and readying us to run or fight. Blood sugar levels rise, serving to increase energy. As the body readies itself for imminent injury, Natural Killer cells are increased in number (preparing to fight infection), and the clotting cascade is initiated (making it easier to stop potential bleeding).

The complement to the sympathetic is the parasympathetic nervous system, which is typified by a relaxed, receptive mode of body and mind. In general, we digest food, store nutrients, engage cellular metabolism (creating energy), and regenerate tissues only to the extent that we are in a parasympathetic mode. Unfortunately, most individuals with chronic illness have spent, and continue to spend, most of their time and energy reserves in a sympathetic nervous system engagement.

The sympathetic mode can be life saving when we need to rapidly mobilize our energies. However, our systems cannot live there for longer than a few minutes at a time without causing some imbalance. With blood moving away from the gut and brain, one cannot digest food or make reasonable decisions. Chronically elevated stress hormones eventually increase insulin production that, in turn, increases the production of LDL cholesterol. The combination of increased peripheral blood pressure, decreased blood to the heart, increased blood clotting, and increased LDL is the perfect combination of factors to cause heart disease.

Stan

I first met Stan when helping his mother through the final stages of cancer. Nine months after her death, Stan came to my office, declaring in his typically affable manner that it was time for him to get on with life. His primary health goal was to recapture a time when he was athletic and felt good about his body. Stan appeared pale and had obviously put on a great deal of weight since I had seen him last. He reported getting short of breath after walking up only one flight of stairs. He had tried to lose weight but failed, and was looking for a diet that he could stick with.

Stan was forty-eight years old and self-employed in a high-stress, time-dependent office job. He was having trouble staying asleep, leaving him to wake tired and needing coffee and cigarettes to get through the day. He had had no sexual partner for some years because of a steadily decreasing libido and, now, a poor body image.

Stan attributed the dramatic diminution in health to the year spent caring for his mother. Even after her demise, he would cook meals reminiscent of a time when the family was whole and happy. Their "comfort foods" consisted of sweets and starches, often mixed with a fat, e.g., bread or baked potatoes with sour cream. Being "a good son," he ate for two, and grew fat.

It concerned Stan that he had lost the hair on his legs and chest during the past year. A physiologic explanation consistent with all of these observations is that Stan was experiencing an increased ratio of estrogen to testosterone. Testosterone regulates the growth of body hair; estrogen regulates head hair. At the same time, carrying extra fat cells, as Stan was about his middle, allows the body to store extra amounts of estrogen. An increased ratio of estrogen to testosterone is also associated with decreased libido.

A physical exam showed that Stan had elevated blood pressure: systolic of 158, diastolic of 100. Most people feel at their best with a systolic between 110 and 130, and a diastolic between 65 and 80. Stan's hypertension was to be expected, given that blood pressure measures the pounds of pressure that must be displaced by the cardiovascular system, and he now had an extra 100 pounds to displace. Even more disturbing was that I could barely detect, with a stethoscope, blood flow through his carotid arteries.

Stan had been to his allopathic physician, who had put him on an anti-hypertensive medication. The drug had effectively lowered blood pressure by about 8 percent, but had also lowered Stan's libido and, with it, his sense of self-worth even more.

The same physician had found elevated cholesterol: Total Cholesterol of 280 and HDL of 52. The ratio of Total to HDL cholesterol was 5.4, certainly an important prognosticator of future cardiovascular disease. Normative statistics indicate that most people have lower incidences of heart disease or atherosclerosis with a ratio of 3.5 or less. Stan's physician prescribed Lovastatin to lower the so-called "bad" low-density (LDL) cholesterol. He counseled that Stan should stop eating cholesterol-rich foods, such as eggs. On questioning, the physician advised (erroneously) that there was nothing to be done to raise the so-called "good" high-density (HDL) cholesterol.

Allopathic medication is sometimes necessary to "stop the bleeding," for example, when the body is too injured to repair itself, but the "tourniquet" must be released before it causes damage of its own. Better still, we should determine, in advance, if a tourniquet is necessary. In Stan's case, we should ask, before medicating him with cholesterol blockers, why his body is producing disproportionately large amounts of LDL cholesterol.

Low-density lipids have the primary function of transporting cholesterol and its derivatives to every cell in the body. The production of cholesterol is essential to life and health: its molecular structure serves as the chemical backbone for the manufacture of all steroid hormones. This includes vitamin D and other hormones produced by the adrenal and reproductive glands. Though seldom discussed, *low* cholesterol levels are hazardous. For example, low cholesterol and correspondingly low hormone levels are associated with *shortened* life span in men and women seventy years of age or older. For the older woman with low cholesterol, there is twice the risk of developing cancer, as well as a mood that she typically describes as "black."

For every biochemical critical to life, there are multiple pathways assuring an optimal level. On average, two-thirds of cholesterol is produced by the liver; the rest is provided by foods we digest. Except for the rare individual born with low numbers of LDL receptors (and therefore cholesterol-starved), eating cholesterol-rich foods causes the liver to produce *less* cholesterol. Given that dietary cholesterol is typically accompanied by fat, it makes biological sense that cholesterol is also essential to the formation of bile salts that digest fats.

On average, one study per month appears in a peer-reviewed medical journal investigating the relationship between egg consumption and serum cholesterol level. There has been very little evidence that eggs elevate LDL cholesterol even in those with high cholesterol levels. In one study, volunteers ate twenty eggs each day for ten days. None of the subjects had a rise in LDL cholesterol, though there was a significant increase in the artery-cleaning HDL. In another experiment, subjects ate two eggs per day for six weeks. Again, HDL rose significantly, while LDL cholesterol remained unchanged except for individuals with low to moderate LDL levels and poor ability to digest fat (i.e., subjects who could use more LDL).

LDL cholesterol is found in clogged arteries, but blaming the former for the latter is like blaming the Dutch boy for obstructing traffic next to the dike. The body uses a cholesterol plaque as mortar to cover scratches in artery walls. Lesions can be caused by any number of things, including infection (e.g., chlamydia), trauma, high homocysteine levels, cancer, or oxidation from high blood sugar. Arterial plaque grows until it breaks, spewing out fat that creates a clot that lodges in the heart (causing a heart attack) or a blood vessel leading to the brain (causing a stroke). A study in the *New England Journal of Medicine* followed 28,000 women for three years, while monitoring their blood values for twelve possible risk factors. LDL cholesterol was not a particularly good predictor of heart disease, heart attack, or stroke. The best marker was an indicator of arterial inflammation in response to a lesion (CRP). The second best predictor was the ratio of HDL to total cholesterol.[1]

Cholesterol is produced in response to an enzyme (HMG CoA Reductase) that is activated by insulin, emotional stress or a rise in stress hormones. As Figure 2.1 (see page 28) depicts, perceived stress is registered by the hypothalamus that presses the pituitary into service, that, in turn, secretes hormonal messages to the thyroid, adrenals, and reproductive glands.

Sustained production of the steroid hormones pregnenolone, adrenaline or cortisol (from the adrenals), or progesterone (from the gonads) demands a lot of cholesterol. A study published January 2001 followed hundreds of men and women, measuring their anxiety levels while analyzing ultrasound images of their carotid arteries. They found that individuals living with daily anxiety had three-and-one-half times more plaque in their arteries than control subjects with only occasional stress.[2]

After more than thirty years of anti-cholesterol prescriptions, there is still no evidence that they increase life span. This should not be surprising if we reflect that the body expends a great deal of energy to maintain optimal cholesterol levels, and that a rise in one's level almost always reflects an increased demand. Such a demand may come from perceived or physiologic stressors, or the need to provide hormones to a body with accelerating growth. As such, we may take an increase in LDL cholesterol level to be symptomatic of the body's changing needs: perhaps emotional stress, an increase in blood glucose, scarring to an artery, increased body fat, or even a tumor.

When Stan came to my office, he had been living with emotional stress for more than two years, meaning that his stress hormones were undoubtedly elevated. With elevated adrenaline or cortisol levels comes insomnia, as the brain is given the message to stay alert, as well as elevated LDL. His increasing number of fat cells made for a diminished libido as well as an additional demand for steroid hormones to produce estrogen.

Stan's complex of health problems were interconnected, creating vicious cycles that were steadily tightening the noose. His care-

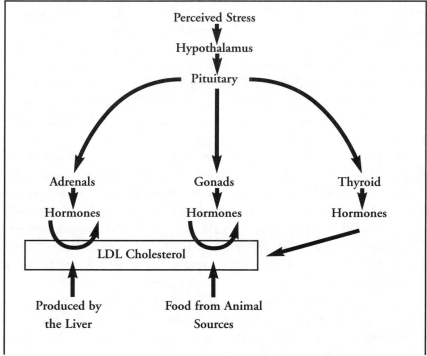

Figure 2.1. Stress hormones supported by LDL cholesterol.

taking duties and time-consuming office job had kept him stressed and not exercising, which, in turn, led to more weight gain, an increased estrogen-to-testosterone ratio, decreased stamina, and diminished ability to extricate himself from the loop. To counteract mental and physical weariness, Stan self-medicated each day with a pack of cigarettes and three cups of coffee, both of which placed more demands on his adrenals, while almost certainly aggravating his hypertension.

While Stan realized that poor management of stress was the cause of his deteriorating health, he saw no way to fundamentally change his lifestyle. "I can't quit my job because I need the money, and I can't exercise because I'm too tired from working." His use of "I can't quit" as an explanation conveniently precludes his looking at options and thereby seems to excuse him from the decision-making process.

Several studies have shown a "Cognitive-Behavioral" approach to be most helpful for dealing with psychosomatic illness. The plan involves challenging or in other ways highlighting the patient's beliefs, assumptions or "shoulds" that prevent him from moving ahead. When such statements are reflected back to the patient, feelings are released along with deeply rooted, often irrational, beliefs that have been unconsciously governing behavior. The therapist's job at this stage is to help the patient recognize the maladaptive nature of those assumptions, often with direct confrontation. The final stage involves helping the patient develop and apply new, more adaptive, behaviors; this is the "working through" that Freud eventually recognized as essential to lasting change, though de-emphasized by classical psychoanalysis.

I asked Stan if he really, literally, meant that maintaining his present job was the only way to make enough money. The answer was, "No, but I just can't do that!" There was, in fact, a modest estate he shared with his sister; it was even possible for him to be more flexible with his work schedule, or to hire someone to assist with the burgeoning workload. But, instead, we had just elicited a deeper (i.e., less approachable) level of "I can't stop..."

"What's the problem Stan?" He answered that his sister blamed him for the poor care of their mother in her final years, and he "certainly could not ask her for money from their estate." "Stan, where was your sister when you were acting as caretaker? Do you really need your sister's approval to access your money?" Stan's affable nature gave way to a look of anger. He was embarrassed by the display of emotion, pointed out that he needed to get back to work, and thanked me on the way out.

It was encouraging that Stan had approached me feeling the need to make a fundamental change in his life. But long-lasting progress would require our dealing with his tendency to escape from unpleasant emotions. At this point I worried that if we couldn't help him to make changes, we would have to resort to allopathic medications just to keep him alive.

During our next consultation, it became clear that Stan felt caught between his allopathic and naturopathic physicians. He felt that he could not initiate a protocol advocated by one without causing disfavor from the other (a form of "I should not..."). In order to reduce the stress accruing from this perceived conflict, I recommended red yeast rice, a natural "statin" (comparable to Lovastatin) shown to help lower inflammatory CRP and LDL. I reminded him that the most effective medications will reduce these values by only 13 percent on average, meaning that it should be understood as support for the changes he was about to make in his lifestyle.

To help with both cholesterol and high blood pressure, and to gently depart from his state of inertia, Stan agreed to get out of his office for a half-hour walk each morning. It is noteworthy that both cholesterol and blood pressure is elevated in *inverse* proportion to the sunlight one receives. Cholesterol is converted into vitamin D in response to ultraviolet light reaching the skin. This, in turn, inhibits production of parathyroid hormone, which, in excess, elevates blood pressure. As Stan developed a tan, he lengthened his walk to an hour.

Besides the walks, Stan began lifting weights in the evenings. I instructed him to use 6-pound dumbbells, flexing and extending them slowly twenty times. I explained that as his strength returned he would be able to lift heavier dumbbells or to lift them slower and slower.

A recent meta-analysis of all experimentally comparable investigations of how exercise affects heart disease found that exercising three times per week is more effective than drugs (such as Digoxin) at preventing heart failure. The researchers also compared "resistance" to "aerobic" workouts for patients recovering from heart failure, finding that weight training causes fewer complications, while producing superior muscle strength and endurance.[3]

For the purposes of burning fat and making muscle, weights are far superior to aerobics. After your heart and respiratory rates recover from an aerobics workout, your metabolism goes into a slow-down period as it gradually returns to a resting state. By comparison, after completing a few minutes of lifting weights, the area of the body being worked continues to burn fat at a high level for the following four hours.

Given all the recommendations, I suggested that it would be best for Stan to decide on his own when to stop smoking. I suggested two possibilities, either of which would help him "come clean" when he was ready to do so: limit the number of cigarettes to under twenty per day, or smoke a pipe with a mixture of natural tobacco and herbs. Stan has chosen to continue smoking cigarettes at about a half-pack per day. Since he periodically reminds me that "sometimes a cigarette is just a cigarette," I, of course, suspect the contrary and look forward to our next discussion around quitting!

I explained that three cups of coffee, while getting him up in the morning, was probably worsening his blood pressure. Probably as a way of pleasing his doctor, Stan immediately switched to green tea, which has less than half the caffeine of coffee and a number of health-giving benefits not found in coffee.

In regards to diet, we needed to make the plan simple. I explained to Stan that when you eat a fat at the same time as a sugar, the body burns the sugar and stores the fat. As a goal, he should become aware of foods high in fat as well as foods that raise one's blood sugar, and then avoid combining them in the same digestive period.

Figure 2.2 lists the Glycemic Index of most common foods. The numbers indicate the extent to which eating a food will raise your blood glucose. While pure glucose has a relative value of 100, sucrose (table sugar) is 75, honey 87, and malt sugar (as found in beer) is 105. A sweet taste does not necessarily come from a food that inordinately raises blood sugar. For example, a yam or sweet potato has half the glycemic index of a white baked potato, the latter being 98 percent as glycemic as pure glucose. Leavened breads

Maltose 105	Parsnips 95
Glucose 100	Carrot juice 87
Honey 95-45	Raw carrots 64-32
Sucrose 75	Beets 75
Fructose 20	Yam 51
	Sweet potato 47
Baked potato 98	
Instant mashed potatoes 98	Leafy Greens 15-5
Boiled potato 70	
	Cantaloupe 65
Puffed rice 95	Pineapple 65
White rice 70	Banana 62
Brown rice 56	Raisins 64
	Grapes 53
	Orange juice 53
White breads 95-72	Orange 42
Whole wheat bread 80-72	Apple juice 40
Pita bread 55	Apple 38
Whole wheat tortilla 55	Grapefruit juice 48
Whole rye bread 50	Grapefruit 25
White pasta 48	Cherries 22
Wild rice 55	Apricots 10
Rye 34	Berries 10
Corn flakes 80	Ice cream 60-36
Shredded Wheat 70	Plain yogurt 36
Grapenuts 65	Whole milk 33
Cream of Wheat 70	
Oatmeal 49	Beans 43-30
Corn chips 75	Lentils 29
Couscous 60	Soybeans 15
Popcorn 55	
Corn 54	Meats (unprocessed) 0

Figure 2.2. Glycemic Index of Some Common Foods.

range from 72 to 95 depending upon how processed they are. In general, the more highly processed the food, the higher the index number. For example, corn flakes are higher than Grapenuts, and white pasta is higher than whole-wheat.

In order to keep it simple, Stan chose to completely avoid some of his comfort foods: leavened bread, flaked cereals, pastry, ice cream, and potatoes (unless eaten alone with salsa). Together we decided that a good breakfast might consist of eggs with spinach and peppers, wrapped in a whole-wheat tortilla. Alternatively, he would enjoy eating oatmeal with berries, a little berry juice for sweetening, with low-fat yogurt and a low-fat milk. He now likes to explore different types of green tea.

As most Americans, Stan eats very little seafood. I explained how a recent study on the dietary practices of medical doctors found that those who ate fish even once per week had half the incidence of heart disease.[4] A couple of easy recipes and the names of inexpensive seafood restaurants got him enjoying fish twice a week.

When you eat a fat at the same time as a sugar, the body burns the sugar and stores the fat.

Besides the red yeast rice, Stan supplemented with 400 IU of vitamin E and 200 mg of Panax ginseng, morning and mid-day. Vitamin E helps prevent harmful oxidation of fatty acids, and lowers inflammatory CRP. Panax is an herb shown to lower blood pressure and LDL, and increase endurance and testosterone levels.

Over the following year, Stan lost 80 pounds, lowered blood pressure to 135/80, and improved Total Cholesterol-to-HDL ratio to 4.0, all without drugs. His libido has returned as a consequence of weight loss and increased muscle, improved flow of blood throughout his vascular system, elimination of hypertensive medication, and an improved body image. His chest hair has returned a little, confirming a stress disorder rather than a "normal" age-related loss of testosterone ("andropause").

Stan will probably always have a need to please. He was even embarrassed to show his allopathic physician that his HDL had increased 20 percent without medication. Contrary to his physician's initial advice, there is excellent evidence that HDL will raise in response to exercise, weight loss, balancing hormones, certain foods and herbs, and stopping smoking.

I can now hear the flow of blood in Stan's carotid arteries, and feel with my fingers a regular pulse on each side of his neck. Of course, progress never takes a straight, level course, but is a sometimes turbulent, sometimes meandering stream; there are even times when one feels better just hiding out in the marshes. Periodically, we talk about those marshes and creating future thoroughfares.

Lilith

With only a cursory look, Lilith appears lean, active, even healthy. However, she feels tired and tearful and very stressed as a night-duty nurse at a local hospital. She has been on and off a variety of medications for high blood pressure, high LDL cholesterol, and low bone density. I showed her to my inner office, where she collapsed into the chair across from my desk.

Being a part of the medical community, Lilith has a great respect for drugs, as well as experience, on a nightly basis, of their dangers. In the U.S., between 76,000 and 137,000 lives are lost each year from properly administered prescription medications, taken as prescribed.[5] Pharmaceutical drugs are therefore ranked, depending upon estimate, from the sixth to the fourth leading cause of death in America. In general, iatrogenic (treatment caused) deaths number approximately 225,000 each year in the U.S., making it the third leading cause of death.[6]

Lilith feels caught between living with her various disorders and taking suppressive drugs along with their side effects. Her blood pressure had been a dangerously high 210/110 until taking clonidine.

Unfortunately, her blood pressure consequently dropped to 102/52, causing lightheadedness and fatigue, while aggravating an already existing tendency to depression. To Lilith's allopathic physician, these effects are all considered "normal" when starting clonidine. When I first saw Lilith, she had unilaterally stopped the clonidine, which had had the effect of raising her blood pressure to 150/80.

Lilith has a combination of symptoms that indicate that she is locked into sympathetic stimulation. She is quite clear that her nightshift hospital work is responsible for her stress, insomnia and fatigue, and is willing to do anything but consider changing her job. "I can't stop now. I am sixty years old, and looking forward to retirement in just five years." I pointed out that when we refuse to stop an unhealthy behavior, our bodies often *make* us stop. I struck a "deal" with Lilith: I would help her regain her health and she would look for daytime work.

Lilith was concerned that her bone density was 20 percent lower than women her age. Two recently published studies, found that, everything else being equal, depressed men and women in their sixties are far more likely to develop osteoporosis. I pointed out to her that the risk is highest for Caucasian women suffering with anxious depression.[7,8]

When stressed, our nervous systems and adrenal glands produce two types of psychoactive regulators (known as "monoamines"): catecholamines such as adrenaline, and long protein chains related to serotonin. Both types of monoamine molecules include magnesium; the catecholamines also demand calcium. No animal has the biochemical resources to live for extended periods in a mode dominated by sympathetic stimulation without cannibalizing its own body. Lilith's body has been leeching magnesium and calcium from its bones in order to handle the stress. Lilith sat up and suggested that the dumping of minerals may be why she has also been suffering from repeated bouts of kidney stones.

The appropriation of one's minerals to service stress happens remarkably fast. For example, an experiment published in *The Journal of Psychosomatic Research* induced excretion of biologically active calcium by causing an agitated state of mind. Adults watched a violent, fast-paced television program intended for children, called *Pokeman*. After twenty minutes their calcium levels were significantly depressed, and remained so for the following two hours. The researchers made the allopathic recommendation that children should drink milk while watching the program![9]

The drug clonidine lowers blood pressure by causing the excretion of the biochemicals that produce the catecholamines that drive the sympathetic nervous system. Patients like Lilith reject such drugs, not because they don't work, but because of how they make them feel. Her body has been cannibalizing itself so as to produce what she needs to cope with her stressors. Suddenly having those chemicals reduced with clonidine without addressing the causes of the stress, left her looking down an abyss.

No animal has the biochemical resources to live for extended periods in a mode dominated by sympathetic stimulation without cannibalizing its own body.

In our discussion of Stan's case, we saw how sunlight can beneficially treat both hypertension and hypercholesterolemia. The production of vitamin D3 in response to ultraviolet light is also essential for laying down bone in a measured way. I asked Lilith how much time she spends out-of-doors, though I could see the answer from her white skin. In her typical day, she would go home after work, fix breakfast, and try to sleep; the rest of the day and early evening was spent with her husband followed by getting ready for the nightshift. On the weekends, she spends most of the day trying to catch up on her sleep.

The lack of sustained, restful sleep aggravates all of Lilith's problems. She knows that she dreams (typically about work!) because she wakes frequently without getting to a deeper level of dreamless sleep. In general, minerals digested from food are stored in the body during deep sleep. This is also the time when minerals dumped into the blood system in response to stress may be restored to the body. Since calcium and magnesium are required for good sleep, Lilith is being pulled down a vicious whirlpool: stress is eating her mineral stores that are necessary for the sleep required to store minerals and recover from the stress. Without addressing the stressors in her life, just taking a mineral supplement will not improve the fundamental situation. This would be like pouring water into a barrel that has holes; you can keep it filled only so long as you continue adding water. At this point I posed the question, "So, how will Lilith change her life so as to patch her barrel?"

Lilith suggested that she would not only look for a day-shift position, but one that she could mentally leave behind at the end of the day. Meanwhile, how do we help restore the sleep "hole," and with which supplements do we refill the "barrel"? Working at night often causes insomnia and related health problems, especially if there are concomitant stressors. It was only three generations ago that most Americans lived in a society where we worked in the sunlight and retired to total darkness for sleep. Today, most of us spend the day inside the house or office with artificial light, which continues via lamps, televisions, and computer monitors, into the night. Even the brightest of tungsten or fluorescent lights is only $1/100,000^{th}$ as bright as a cloudy day. The perpetual twilight in which most of us live is far from the sharp contrast of light and darkness from which we evolved, and we pay the price.

We have evolved a hormonal system that functions at an optimal level when we get sunlight twelve to thirteen hours before bedtime. This signals the pineal gland, located at the rear of the brain's center for emotions and between the branches of the optic nerve, to start storing melatonin to assist in that night's sleep. In the summer time, Lilith will make a point of getting sunlight from 6 to 7 P.M. (twelve to thirteen hours before her bedtime); at other times of the year, it might be necessary to use a full-spectrum sunlamp. Astronauts on long voyages require daily periods of sunlamp exposure to maintain their wake-sleep cycles and avoid depression.

Studies show that men and women working a night shift are

helped to sleep by taking melatonin at the hour of sleep. As with other hormones, it is best to start at a low dose and work up as needed: 0.5 mg may be sufficient and is available as part of an herbal tea.

The release of melatonin is inhibited if there is so much as one candle flame of light in one's bedroom. Lilith will need to shore-up her bedroom so as to insulate it from any light when she goes to bed. I explained that it might be best to spend thirty to sixty minutes in the dark before sleeping. Like many other patients told this, Lilith wondered what there was to do for thirty minutes in the dark! I reminded her that this was one of the few times in the day when she could luxuriate in the parasympathetic mode: meditate, listen to music, make love, or just be; she could even listen to a book on tape. Lilith responded by asking if she should just take higher doses of melatonin, and I pointed out that with hormones more is not better.

We have evolved a hormonal system that functions at an optimal level when we get sunlight twelve to thirteen hours before bedtime.

Besides melatonin, I prescribed calcium (300 mg hydroxyapatite) and 600 mg magnesium citrate to supply the demand for stress hormones, and flush-free niacin (600 mg inositol-hexaniacinate) to help lower LDL, raise HDL, and promote sustained sleep. These supplements were to be taken with Lilith's nighttime meal.

All the minerals you can digest will not lay down strong bone unless it serves the body's needs. Weight-bearing exercise is essential to stopping and reversing osteoporosis. When you use your muscles, blood pumps through the area, making way for larger muscles, which, in turn, gives the message to the body to produce larger bones for support. A number of studies published the past three years have shown how bone loss can be reversed by doing weight ("resistance") training. In one study, ten minutes per day for eight weeks significantly increased muscle strength and bone density in post-menopausal women.[10] Another study found 15 to 20 minutes, only twice per week, to reverse osteoporosis. Lilith agreed to lift 4-pound dumbbells, 20 repetitions at a time, every other day.[11]

Often, when it seems we have grasped the essence of a case, we find that we've just shed one layer. How healthy was Lilith before working night shifts? I asked her: "Suppose we were in a balloon looking down on Lilith as a little girl. What would we see? Would I recognize you in a school photo?" She answered, "I think I look the same: still thin, still running." On reflection, she had always had a tendency to anxious depression, with a "fix-it" disposition.

Stressful situations had always affected her menstrual periods, prolonging them or making them not appear at all. Her last period had been at age thirty-one. Her gynecologist speculated that the early menopause might have been caused by a problem in the hypothalamus. Lilith, at least at sixty, did not attach much significance to this event, and recalls having felt "relieved by no longer having periods."

With a history of chronic stress affecting both the adrenal and reproductive glands, the problem is most certainly at the level of the hypothalamus or pituitary. The hypothalamus is a small gland located in the brain at a point central to the sense organs, beneath the emotional centers, and above the brain stem which regulates basic functions such as blood pressure. It sends chemical messages down to the pituitary in response to perceived changes in the internal or external environment. In turn, the pituitary sends chemical messages to the adrenal, thyroid, or reproductive glands. While the hypothalamus acts as an appraiser and prioritizer, the pituitary is the "budget officer" allotting certain amounts of energy to each of the subsidiary glands.

"Lilith, it sounds as though you've never stopped running. Thirty years ago, your body redirected its energy from reproduction to adrenals in order to keep you going. More recently, you've been fueling that energy by combusting your bones, and now, with a nightshift, you're feeling the enervation." That was quite a mouthful, but she got the message.

She wanted to know if I thought she could survive another five years. Despite the elevated blood pressure, her pulses were weak. This was especially the case with the wrist pulse identified in Oriental medicine as "Kidney Yin," corresponding to one's reservoir of energy. On the other hand, her "Kidney Yang" pulse felt irregular and frantic, suggesting that her remaining energy was being marshaled to keep her awake. "In my opinion, you can choose to rest or soon have your body force it upon you. If you choose to wait, you will eventually suffer adrenal exhaustion, when it will take longer for you to recover."

This is one of those situations when the physician realizes that everything is now in the hands of the patient. Fortunately, Lilith decided to take some vacation time to rest. We added to her protocol (a) bovine adrenal cortex to allopathically restore adrenal nutrients, and (b) phosphorylated L-Serine, an amino acid that serves as a neurotransmitter and assists to reprogram the hypothalamus and pituitary.

Lilith felt a healthful vigor returning over the ensuing months. Pulses on each wrist are now regular and balanced. Her blood pressure has decreased without the use of pharmaceutical drugs to a "borderline high" 135/75, while her ratio of total cholesterol to HDL is a close-to-ideal 3.7. After only six months of weight training, Lilith's bone density improved to being slightly superior to that of the average sixty-year-old.

Eight months after starting to turn things around, Lilith found a daytime nursing position. Between jobs, she took two weeks off, during which time she got morning sunlight and weaned herself from melatonin. Since, with the new job, she is able to spend more "quality time" with her husband, she is experiencing greater health in both "love" and "work." She appears to enjoy more hours in deep sleep, waking more rested, feeling more vital. Everything feels easier to accomplish.

Lilith has always liked the feeling of being "charged up." Now that she feels more energy, she is considering resuming the night shift on a part-time basis. On telling me this, she observed my disappointment and her smile became more enigmatic (the left half oddly resembling that of Dali's *Madonna*). I reminded her that inertia is a powerful force that grows so long as one chooses to nurse its existence. Her real challenge will be holding the new course after so many years living with sympathetic nervous system overdrive.

Richard

There are people who understand how they get themselves into trouble, but just can't stop; or, knowing what they need to do, can't hold the course in the face of the inevitable challenges life presents. Reflecting on failed attempts makes one lose confidence in his or her ability to make meaningful changes, and steadily feeds the vicious cycle of depression.

Richard is a forty-nine-year-old massage therapist, who has suffered on and off for most of his life with clinical depression, anxious depression and obsessive thinking. "I'm always doing things to throw myself out of balance. And all the medications I'm taking make me feel unreal." Richard's assertion "I can't stop making myself depressed" is based on a long history of therapies that have failed to support behavior conducive to a healthy mind. Because of this, he maintains a stable of health-care practitioners to answer questions regarding the best therapies for him: a psychiatrist, primary care medical doctor, chiropractor, acupuncturist, counselor, psychic, yoga instructor, and, now, a naturopathic physician. Of course, each therapist has a different perspective, and, lacking a strong sense of self, Richard finds himself spinning more and more out of control. The inability of Richard's practitioners to help also stems from the fact that it is impossible to listen and make reasonable decisions when depressed.

There is some confusion as to the term "depression." It is used at one time or another by most of us to describe feeling down or "blue." But, *clinical depression* is rarely seen by the public, or even by a primary care physician. It involves the diminution of life-sustaining functions, including eating and sleeping; the depressed person often feels "numb" and is generally not motivated to communicate. All of this prevents one from working and loving. By contrast, *anxious depression* is a persistent anxiety disorder, characterized by sympathetic nervous system overdrive that taxes one's energy reserves. One can still love and work, but has a growing apprehension that that ability will be lost. Unlike clinical depression, the patient is tormented by his feelings and motivated to end the anxiety. Anxious depression from which one can see no way out may lead to suicide.

How does one get to the point of hanging over an emotional abyss? Almost always this involves living with a stressful situation that one feels helpless to change. It may be in the workplace, or a personal relationship, or as a victim in a supercharged environment controlled by terrorists.

The physical consequences of living in a controlled environment are immediate and profound. A number of studies have measured physical parameters in a captive audience of medical students.[12] In general, total cholesterol, adrenaline, blood pressure, and blood glucose rise significantly (8 to 33 percent) during times of extreme stress, e.g. during an important examination. One found that at times of relatively low stress (between examinations), blood cholesterol averaged 205. This in itself is abnormally high, given a population of young, mostly healthy men and women. But, during finals week, cholesterol levels rose 10 percent to an average of 226. Since this training is intended as preparation for professional life, it is no wonder that medical doctors are more likely to die of cerebrovascular disease than is the population they treat.

Of course, medical students have been pre-selected to be competitive in a structured environment. A 1993 meta-analysis of "Type A" personalities found that their heart rates and blood pressures rose significantly more than others when being evaluated or criticized. Type A individuals are twice as likely to have heart disease as those who are more laissez faire.[13]

For people harboring hostility, the situation is even worse: five to six times the risk of heart disease as has the general population. Hostility can manifest as (a) the belief that others are untrustworthy, incompetent, deceitful or selfish, (b) feelings of irritability, impatience or hatred, or (c) the aggressive acting out of anger. As you might imagine, physicians, attorneys, and other high-stress professionals living with these feelings are five times as likely as their more laid-back colleagues to die by age fifty.

Richard, while not particularly competitive, does feel trapped in his present work and love relationships, harbors hostility toward everyone around him, and suffers, above all else, that he is impotent to alter his situation. This is a vicious whirlpool pulling him steadily downward toward clinical depression. In the past, it has led to his hospitalization.

During the past two years, Richard's psychiatrist has experimented with having him take various combinations of drugs. Patients like Richard will typically take a medication to manage the anxiety as long as it does not deplete their energy. Unfortunately, the new generation of anti-anxiety medications suppresses the catecholamine pathway and, in so doing, makes the patient feel deprived of the energy he uses to cope with stress. Alternatively, there are drugs that promote the serotonin or GABA brain pathways, each of which serves to relax the body and mind. GABA stimulators, like Valium or Xanax, are intended to relax you when in the midst of a panic attack, or in anticipation of a high stress situation. Their manufacturers clearly indicate that the drugs have only been found safe and efficacious when taken situationally or for no more than a few weeks at a time. Despite these warnings, physicians are likely to put an anxious patient on such a drug indefinitely or until problems arise.

Drugs can force a patient's body into a parasympathetic mode, and this might be life preserving. But, if the patient is still facing real stressors, the body will soon start modifying itself to compensate for the drugs; for example, within days, receptors along the catecholamine pathway will start multiplying or becoming more sensitive. Once the nervous system has been altered, the patient is again "free" to experience tormenting anxiety. It is this physiologic adaptation that psychiatric researchers cite for not trusting the long-term efficacy of low-dose medications. Psychiatrists who feel impotent to help patients deal meaningfully with their stress are likely to use the phenomenon of drug tolerance as the rationale for prescribing a "tourniquet" to the patient's nervous system at a dose stronger than is initially necessary.

As a naturopathic physician, I am interested in how Richard's body is adapting to his various stressors. There are two biochemical pathways that address emotional stressors by producing complementary hormones. The catecholamines are produced in the brain, sympathetic nerve endings, and the adrenal glands. The process begins with the amino acid phenylalanine (the richest natural source being soft cheese) or L-tyrosine (most concentrated in shellfish), and ends with the storage of adrenaline ("epinephrine").

The B-vitamin folic acid is essential for the conversion of L-tyrosine to L-dopa. One means by which caffeine speeds us up is by accelerating this conversion. The very same biochemical conversion occurs in beans when they are baked!

Vitamin B-6 is essential to the production of dopamine from L-dopa, and vitamin C is essential to noradrenaline ("norepinephrine") production. Finally, adrenaline is produced from noradrenaline and the amino acid methionine (found richly in seafood and sunflower seeds).

Noradrenaline and adrenaline molecules are conjoined with magnesium and calcium and stored in the inner recesses of the adrenal glands. A number of drugs produce a sympathetic nervous system "high" by preventing our reservoir of noradrenaline and adrenaline from being digested by the enzyme monoamine oxidase (MAO). Cocaine (one of Freud's anti-depressants), kava-kava, imipramine, Marplan, Nardil, and other related drugs, serve to maintain these hormones, and thereby elevate mood.

A complementary biochemical pathway, one that promotes the parasympathetic nervous system, is that leading to the production of serotonin and its derivatives. Serotonin has many bodily functions, including sleep, digestion, and pain reduction. The vitamin and essential amino acid L-tryptophan is converted into niacin, and (in conjunction with folic acid, vitamin B-6 and magnesium) into 5-hydroxytryptophan (5-HTP). Contrary to "medical gossip,"consuming turkey or milk will not raise your levels of tryptophan unless you are generally protein deficient. The most concentrated food source of

L-tryptophan is lager beer. One may prejudice the conversion of L-tryptophan away from niacin and toward serotonin by supplementing with niacin (thereby reducing the body's need to produce it) and by avoiding competing amino acids (e.g., those in milk, millet, or molasses).

The conversion from L-tryptophan to serotonin is facilitated by chromium. Even modest amounts of chromium picolinate (400 mcg) significantly increase serotonin levels in the brain and reduce anxious depression. Serotonin is actually found in certain foods, most notably in eggplant and pineapple. But, the most controlled means of raising serotonin involves taking its immediate precursor, 5-HTP.

Short-term use of the herb St. John's Wort (*hypericum*) increases the number of serotonin receptors[14] and is, therefore, a good combination with 5-HTP. By contrast, long-term use of hypericum reduces all stress hormones, including serotonin, dopamine, noradrenaline, and GABA.[15] This makes it, like Serzone and Zyprexa, appropriate for someone suffering from manic-depressive mood swings (bipolar disorder). Using hypericum for longer than thirty days has also been found to relieve depression as efficaciously as imipramine, though with less likelihood of causing anxiety.[16]

Richard has taken these and other psychoactive drugs, with no relief from anxious depression for longer than a few days at a stretch. Over the years he has accumulated a war-chest of prescription drugs and over-the-counter nutraceuticals, and tries various combinations every few days. This is, of course, dangerous, and the consequence of having a string of physicians (myself included), each attempting to ease his suffering without addressing the role Richard plays in perpetuating his anxiety. I contacted Richard's psychiatrist, who agreed to store his stash of drugs. Henceforth, he was to use only one drug: 0.5 mg Xanax, as needed.

Most people who rely on pills for their state of well being also use food, sex or other behaviors to self-medicate. When feeling "down," Richard indulges in high glycemic foods (bread and pastry), which yields a short-term rush that is inevitably followed by more depression. He also uses sex as a way of releasing tension, which soon thereafter makes him feel vulnerable and "weak."

Richard cannot stop worrying about his condition and the proper combination of medicinals. He cannot stop depending upon his health-care practitioners to make decisions for him. He cannot stay asleep, eat without getting indigestion, or work or make love without feeling fatigued. Richard's sensitivity and boyish good looks are attractive to women, though he can maintain a romantic relationship only to the extent that the woman is committed to nursing his disorder. He is tormented by his inability to alter course the way he knows he should, and by the prospect of "never being normal."

Richard despises most people for being incompetent, but not nearly so much as he despises himself. He beats-up on himself for self-destructive behavior that ranges from ordering a difficult-to-digest food because it is liked by his companion, to moving from a city he loved because he couldn't bear running into an ex-girlfriend.

"Richard, it all sounds hopeless and horribly depressing."

He did not approve of this comment, "You're not supposed to tell me that; I need hope."

I summarized his past two years of therapies saying, "Despite the best efforts of all your practitioners, you seem to be suffering more and more."

Richard has always resisted the inference that meaningful changes will come only from him, and countered with a typical deflection, "I know if I could only see the Dalai Lama's physician, he could give me the herbs I need."

"Richard, are you really so optimistic that there are special herbs known to the Dalai Lama's personal physician that would fix you, and that he would give you a consultation?"

"Why are you doing this to me today. My chiropractor never talks to me like that." His voice was coming in short gasps. I explained, "We need to do things differently. For example, today I'm not going to answer any question that we've discussed before. Today is for reflection and relaxation."

I felt Richard's wrist pulses. In general they were weak though rapid. If you take enough pulses and blood pressures, you learn to read the latter from the former. Richard's blood pressure typically runs low (about 110/70). I recommend to all healthcare practition-ers that they feel their patient's pulses at both wrists, ankles and carotid arteries. This tells directly if there is an imbalance between the left and right sides or between the upper and lower torsos. With some practice, one can read the moment-to-moment changes in a pulse corresponding to changes in the patient's blood flow, chem-istry or mood.

The pulse is the primary diagnostic tool in the traditional Oriental medicines. Going to a traditional Chinese doctor is often referred to as "going to have my pulses felt." The tips of one's index, middle and ring fingers are gently placed around the patient's radi-al artery at the wrist. The middle finger is placed on the *radial emi-nence* (at the middle wrist crease), with the other fingers almost touching either side (and close to the other wrist creases). If your hand is smaller than that of the patient's, then you will need to spread the fingers slightly to compensate. After a few seconds, you will notice that the pulse feels different under each finger. Gently press each pulse in turn and note how the pulse responds. Next, using your other hand, turn your attention to the patient's other wrist. Again, notice differences in relative strength, size and respon-siveness of each pulse.

During the past ten years, the scientific method has begun to be applied to the study of pulse diagnosis. It has now been confirmed, for example, that most patients suffering from heart disease have a

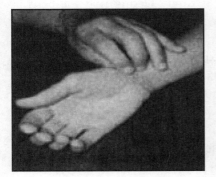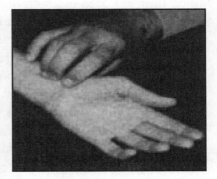

Figure 2.3. A patient has her pulses read.

thin, "string-like" pulse, and that this is due to reduced amounts of blood being ejected each contraction, reduced flexibility in the arteries, and increased peripheral blood pressure. It has been confirmed that patients with an infection have a rapid, string-like *Pitta* pulse that moves away under finger pressure.[17] This is due to increased pumping action of the heart, a shortened ejection period each heart contraction and lowered peripheral blood pressure.

When people feel most balanced their pulses are equally strong, robust, and responsive. In Ayurvedic medicine, the three wrist pulses extending up the arm indicate the state of *Vata*, *Pitta*, and *Kapha*, respectively. When Richard is hysterical, his *Vata* pulse is highly reactive, meaning that it changes rhythm and frequency within only a few seconds of light pressure, and changes location in response to greater pressure. At such times, his *Pitta* (or digestive) pulse is weak and disappears on pressure. Since in sympathetic system overdrive one's ability to digest is minimal, even the healthiest foods will cause Richard indigestion. Meanwhile, his *Kapha* pulse cannot be felt at all. This pulse lies deeper under the fascia of the arm, and therefore requires a good amount of blood displacement to be felt strongly. In the Chinese system of pulse diagnosis, the *Kapha* pulse corresponds to the kidneys and fluid balance. Someone who is dehydrated or with low blood pressure will have weak pulses at this deeper level.

Richard lay down and I applied acupuncture needles to his ankles and wrists so as to stimulate *Kapha*/kidney energy (Ki-3) and calm *Vata* hysteria (P-7). As he lay there I started a hypnotic induction. I asked him to "Become aware of that tingly feeling that happens as your muscles just let go. Perhaps it will be your feet or calves…or the front of your thighs, as they just let go. You might just wonder which part of your body will give that relaxing, tingly feeling next…though it may not be time for you to relax your eyes quite yet…Relaxing without knowing at times how much more comfortable you can become…Perhaps your butt…or lower abdomen…or your shoulders and upper back will feel that pleasant tingly sensation…You can feel your upper arms or your hands just let go…Perhaps, the back of your neck…or your face and eyes…up to even your scalp letting go."

Here I watched his breathing as it became deeper and slower, and guided him into a deeper hypnotic trance with imagery I knew to be conducive to Richard's relaxation. "The sound of my voice, the sound of your breath, even the feeling of breath on your face, are just like ripples on a pond; a pebble dropping into a sun-drenched lake…One ripple, then another, spreading out and out as the pebble slowly sinks into the water…You might look up and see the sunlight filtering through the water and the ripples spreading ever thinner, as you go deeper…Or you can look down and feel the water gently caressing and gently turning you. You need not proceed too fast all at once…but wonder where your mind will take you next." At this point, I allowed Richard to enjoy the hypnagogic state for a few minutes.

"In a few moments, but not until you are ready to do so, you will begin to become aware again of the world around you." Notifying someone in trance that the session is coming to an end often leads to an even deeper level, perhaps because they very much enjoy the experience. A couple of minutes later, I reminded Richard that "When you are ready, you will be floating up through the water…gently…becoming more and more aware of the light filtering down from above, the sounds about you…your own breathing. You will remember how well this feels, and know that you can return here whenever you want." About three minutes later, Richard began to stir, when I surprised him with the information that he had been relaxing for the past twenty minutes.

After removing the needles, I took Richard's pulses again. For the first time, I felt his pulses in all six positions to be balanced and regular and gently pushing against my fingers. Still in a parasympathetic glow, his face looked relaxed and his voice sounded deeper.

Richard and I have worked out a program that feels right to him: (a) strictly avoiding caffeine, dairy, shellfish, sugar, molasses, white bread and pastry, (b) 0.5 mg Xanax, as needed, (c) a vitamin B-complex (including niacin and folic acid) each morning, (d) a mineral supplement with magnesium, calcium, and chromium picolinate each night, (e) 200 mg 5-HTP and 300 mg hypericum before lunch and before bed, (f) a vigorous walk in the sunlight each morning (protecting eyes and skin in the afternoon), (g) practice laughing to the point of tears (*Pink Panther* movies do the trick). Perhaps most importantly, he practices self-hypnosis every morning. This gives him the sense that he can control his mind without looking to others for approval.

Over the past four months, Richard has scaled down his stable of practitioners, and rarely needs the Xanax. The best news from him has come in the form of a postcard from Crater Lake: "Having a good time. Glad you're not here!"

Louis

The inability to stop can manifest at various levels. Sometimes cells of the body grow without stopping, thus producing warts, endometriosis, benign tumors, or cancers. Cancer cells are immature cells that lack the genetic programming necessary to mature and die. Louis has made an appointment to see me, having just been told by his oncologist that he has Stage 3 pancreatic cancer. This means that a tumor with highly undifferentiated (immature) cells has been detected growing in his pancreas and surrounding lymph nodes, though it has not as yet spread (metastasized) to other areas. He is scheduled to begin the first round of chemotherapy and is interested in alternative therapies. His immediate concern is not offending his oncologist by appearing to question her judgment.

We might suppose that a patient, upon hearing that he or she has an advanced stage of cancer, would be highly motivated to make life-preserving changes. Unfortunately, this is rarely the case. Individuals who develop a cancerous tumor more often than not have a pattern of appeasing others while denying their own needs. Such patients lack the psychosocial skills to fight the disease. While the behavior pattern has undoubtedly existed for many years, it becomes immediately obvious on entering the oncologist's waiting room. Patients appear stunned and to have suspended all critical thought. Clinical hypnotists advise that there is no need to do a formal hypnotic induction for patients who see their lives to be in the doctor's hands. In a hypnagogic state, patients are likely to turn a comment, even an incidental one, into a prescription. The implications are obvious: anyone interacting with a patient who feels vulnerable should be aware of the suggestions they impart.

Unfortunately, since Louis' oncologist believes that patient compliance is necessary for survival, she tells each of her new patients that they "will suffer and eventually die unless they follow the proven therapy." What the cancer patient *hears* is that he or she *will die a horrible death*, and that *making decisions on one's own behalf will make matters even worse.*

Anyone interacting with a patient who feels vulnerable should be aware of the suggestions they impart.

Many studies have found that cancer patients who exhibit a fighting spirit have a more favorable outcome. But, it is not sufficient to simply describe this phenomenon to individuals who have spent their lives avoiding conflict. Even if you suggest that they need to be more assertive, they are likely to simply agree with you! Society conspires to reinforce malleable behavior. Those in positions of authority are supportive of self-deprecating behavior, while disdaining attempts at self-assertion. For example, doctors dislike dealing with feisty patients, and often quip, "Why is it the (*explicative deleted*) who lives the longest?"

"Louis, being told that you have cancer must be frightening." He shook his head, puckered his lips, closed his eyes, and said, "Oh, you can't let things bother you." He looked up and his smile returned. I asked "Do you feel any pain?" Louis answered, "No, I feel fine, just some nausea. Of course I don't like the idea of chemotherapy; I understand that you can give me some herbs that will help."

I decided to begin by addressing Louis' overt request. "Your body is fighting for its life, and it will help if you implement a number of changes. There are, for example, some herbal formulas that will make the chemotherapy safer and even more effective." At this point in the discussion, Louis looked relieved. I continued, "Before prescribing some herbs, we will need to know more about you as an individual. The traditional Chinese or Japanese herbalist tailors the herbal formula to the individual. Each person is different in his metabolism, in what has caused his cancer, in his social support network, and what he is willing to do to fight the cancer." From his face, I could tell that Louis had just slipped into a light trance.

Louis exhibits all the characteristics of Type C behavior: denial or suppression of emotions (especially anger), avoiding conflict, and overly compliant behavior. These behavior patterns are prevalent in patients with any form of cancer. Moreover, the more pronounced these behaviors, the more virulent is the cancer.

A meta-analysis of forty-six studies investigating the relationship between psychosocial factors and breast cancer found the most significant psychosocial predictor of breast cancer to be the use of denial or repression as a way of managing stress.[18] This was closely followed in statistical significance by there having been, prior to tumor detection, a recent death or loss of a loved one. Also found to be statistically significant were "living with chronic stress" and "a pattern of conflict avoidance." From similar studies we know that colorectal cancer is more common in those who have had an unhappy life while feeling unable to discuss their anxiety.

Of all the factors that contribute to the development of breast cancer, *the* most significant was recently discovered and published in the journal *Cancer* (2001).[19] Price, et al, found that women experiencing a high level of stress without intimate emotional support have nine times the risk of developing breast cancer as women with such support. So powerful are the effects of a loving partner or confidant that they can erase the damage caused by highly threatening stressors or a Type C personality. I have no doubt that this relationship is just as true for men, as well as for other types of cancer.

The healing ability of intimacy applies equally well to the cardiovascular system. One study followed 10,000 men for five years, observing the emergence of angina and heart disease.[20] Even when there was a combination of physical and psychosocial risk factors, there was one half the incidence of heart pain in men who viewed their wives as emotionally supportive. Subsequent studies have found that a spouse who makes solicitous words in response to heart disease symptoms actually worsens the condition,[21] while loving support that rebuilds the patient's esteem speeds recovery.[22] Even animals reap cardiovascular benefits from being stroked. In one double-blind experiment, rabbits randomly assigned to be "lovingly stroked" once a day developed only half the fatty deposits in their arteries as normally treated rabbits.

One thing the Type A and Type C individuals have in common is that they can both become healthy with regular loving strokes.

To health-care practitioners I advise asking their patients what makes them angry. Patients who answer by gritting their teeth and displaying obvious signs of frustration and hostility, are at increased risk for heart disease. If, on the other hand, they answer with a socially acceptable chuckle, shake of the head or verbal downplaying of the question's significance (e.g., "That's just life") then they are at increased risk for cancer. One thing the Type A and Type C individuals have in common is that they can both become healthy with regular loving strokes.

I asked Louis how his wife is doing with the news of his pancreatic cancer. "She is always so thoughtful and busy working that I can't bear to dump this on her." I immediately called our local cancer center's support group, and encouraged Louis to take in the next meeting. I explained, "Only by taking care of yourself will you be able to help those who love you." He thought his wife, Patricia, might be able to come with him for our next consultation.

On subsequent visits I obtained a more complete look at Louis' health, often with the help of Patricia. At one time or another, medical specialists had diagnosed Louis with Peyronies disease (tightened fibers of the penis, making erections painful), and hemorrhoids believed to have developed from tightening muscles during intercourse so as to prevent ejaculation. By the time Patricia reminded Louis of his chronically "frozen shoulder" (stiff and painful to move), he could only muster a chuckle at the many ways in which he holds himself in.

Louis had been a drinking alcoholic when he and Patricia met. In fact, at that time, she had been most attentive to his needs. After a drink or two, Louis would open up—laugh passionately, cry and show his vulnerability. He hadn't thought of himself as an alcoholic until overhearing a conversation in the men's bathroom, in which he was described as "one of the those fun-to-watch drunks." He quietly walked out of the bar and never drank again. I complemented him for having the fortitude to stay sober the past thirty years. Past successes remind one that he or she has the ability to overcome existing problems.

Alone, I asked Louis if he knew where those uninhibited tears are now. He shook his head and looked away. "Louis, imagine that we're up in a blimp, looking at you as a young child. Describe what we would see."

"I was just a normal boy."

I asked him to focus on his image. "Would I recognize you in a school photo from your first or second grades?"

"Yes, I think so. I was tall and thin; I pretty much looked the same as today."

I expanded the image: "Would we see other people with you, as we looked down from the blimp? What would you be doing?"

"Outside, running around, usually with other kids."

I commented, "That sounds like a normal, happy picture of a child. I guess you laughed and cried just like other normal children. Suppose we focus the blimp's telescope onto a time when that child was laughing or crying."

"Of course, this is all the past, and it doesn't really matter any more, does it?"

I recognized Louis' response as a half-hearted attempt at deflection, and replied, "Well, some events don't matter and others don't not matter. Since you don't cry now, but did as a child, I was wondering what has changed?"

"Real men don't cry," he stated matter-of-factly, his eyes peering through his eyebrows.

I felt myself smiling, but exerted enough control to ask, "Which frame of your life are we looking at that says real men don't cry?"

He laughed succinctly and then shared that his "father loved John Wayne movies." After a few moments of quiet, he continued, his voice sounding choked up. "My mother was afraid that any noise would disturb him. If I cried, she would beat me until I stopped."

"Louis, *my* eyes are as wet as yours! One more question. Was your father alcoholic?"

"Of course he was," Louis responded with a sigh.

"And aren't you angry as hell?"

"My father was just an old drunk that people liked to make fun of…Sort of like me."

"You *were* a drunk but changed that. How do you feel about your mother?"

"I hated her, but got over that."

"Unfortunately, Louis, we have to work through these issues *each* time we mature."

Louis has obviously been living in an emotional purgatory. Since he appears afraid of what his feelings may reveal ("I dare not stop being a child"), I decided to give him some breathing room by putting on my physician's "cap." I addressed the question forming on Louis' face: "I'll bet you're wondering how all this is going to help you recover from cancer. For one thing, each moment that you are in touch with your feelings, your immune system gets a boost."

One technique for studying *psychoneuroimmunology* (the relationship between state of mind, the nervous system, and the immune system) is to continually monitor blood values while having subjects do things that modify their mood.[23,24] In one such study, subjects were asked to recall a time when they felt loved. The result was that, within seconds, immune system blood markers were increased by about 50 percent. In another experiment, survivors of the San Francisco earthquake were asked to write about their experience while their blood count was being monitored. Again, dealing with feelings (in this case trauma) effectively boosted all immune markers in real time. We should note that no substance at any price, natural or synthetic, can improve immune function as much as *feeling*. On the other hand, anger swallowed, or the numbness that accompanies depression, gives the immune system the dangerous message that one is not worth protecting.

In regards to Louis' request for "herbs that will help with chemotherapy," I recommended that he drink four cups of tea each day, and to eat foods rich in the bioflavonoid quercetin (e.g., cooked onions, black or oolong tea). Both green tea and quercetin prevent the body from becoming resistant to chemotherapeutic agents, thus allowing for longer drug schedules at lower, and safer, doses. Green tea also enhances the effects of various chemotherapies, increasing the drug's concentration in cancer cells by a factor of 2.5, while protecting normal cells.[25]

Over the past thirty years, Chinese and Japanese researchers have systematically tested the efficacy of traditional herbal formulations in conjunction with conventional therapies. Astragalus root and Panax (ginseng) root are the most common of the herbs included in these formulas, each of which has been individually tested for its cancer fighting ability. Research on human cells shows that Panax increases the concentration of chemotherapeutic agents within cancer cells by selectively altering the cancer cell membrane so as to prevent the drug from escaping into healthy tissue.[26]

As a complement to chemotherapy, I also recommended that he take each morning 200 mg natural vitamin E and a tablespoon of fish oil (when not actually eating fish). A study published in the journal *Cancer* found that the combination helps to extend life in those with advanced cancers by increasing the proportion of T-Helper cells.[27] Vitamin E has also been found in numerous animal experiments to mitigate adverse side effects of chemotherapeutic agents, while increasing their anti-tumor activity.

Since one of the pancreas' primary functions is digestion, it is important to facilitate digestion via salivary and stomach enzymes, and by eating fresh, lightly cooked foods. When pancreas function is compromised, as in pancreatic cancer, indigestion and nausea are sure to follow. Fresh ginger grated into warm water stimulates the release of digestive enzymes and reduces nausea. It has been found to be as effective as pharmaceutical drugs in managing nausea from seasickness, morning sickness, or chemotherapy.

The most important change in diet will be the elimination of all highly glycemic foods. While managing blood glucose levels is helpful for all cancer patients, it is essential to those with pancreatic cancer. The pancreas is the organ responsible for producing the insulin to metabolize glucose; however, the disease and the chemotherapy will increasingly tax its function. Louis' blood glucose levels have been borderline high for many years, though they rose sharply recently, in part because his insulin production is compromised. Here is a vicious cycle based on the fact that glucose is the favorite fuel of cancer cells: replacement of pancreatic islets by cancer cells decreases insulin production, which maintains high glucose levels, which promotes cancer reproduction.

Controlling his sugar intake will be a challenge, since, like many reformed alcoholics, Louis craves sweets. I explained that if he ate only low glycemic foods for the next three days, his craving would diminish. After that, his prescribed herbs will help manage his blood sugar if he happens to eat white potatoes, bread, sugar, or white rice. By drinking green tea with meals and taking a Panax capsule forty minutes to an hour before meals, glucose levels are less likely to spike.

I reminded Louis that beyond the drugs, herbs and dietary support, the best predictor of success is whether the cancer patient, supported by his loved ones, is determined to make fundamental changes. Louis reflected, "I spent years making cells that never grow up." I asked what *his* growing up will mean. He answered, "It will mean speaking out. Speaking my mind without being afraid of what someone will think." I asked what was in his heart right now. With tears and a smile, Louis answered, "I'm frightened to death, almost."

Louis survived four sessions of chemotherapy, six weeks of group psychotherapy, and a brief separation from Patricia. Four years later, he is more aware than ever of anxiety or anger as the feelings arise. He is now more likely to stand up to controlling personalities. He is also more aware of his feelings of love and the love coming from others. To the oncologist, the cancer is nearly in remission. Louis explains his health by saying, "With all that I feel going on inside me, I have no more room for cells that won't grow up."

CHAPTER THREE

Never Well Since...

A life may be described as having been "never well since..."
when a stressful event demarcates the beginning of a chronically diminished state of health. Such events may directly
affect one's physical state of health or act as a temporal landmark
that anchors one to an illness. The following case illustrates how
one's life-skills can be used to navigate the medical system and thereby overcome a life threatening disease.

In the summer of 1964, Norman Cousins was an editor at
Saturday Review and diplomat to the Soviet Union. Having worked
for a month to start a dialogue on cultural exchange, Mr. Cousins
had grown fatigued. His final night in Moscow was meant as the
culmination of his delegation's efforts at détente. Instead, his State-
appointed chauffeur delivered him to the *dacha* four hours late and

"frazzled." At the airport the next morning he felt as though events had slipped out of his control, and by the time exhaust fumes of a nearby jet hit him "at point-blank range" he was already feeling feverish and achy.

Within days after returning home, Cousins was examined, and found to have a steadily increasing sedimentary rate, a blood test that indirectly measures inflammation. The achiness in his joints steadily deepened. The diagnosis was rheumatoid (aka *ankylosing*) spondylitis, a chronic inflammatory joint disease. The disease begins with an infection or other stressor that triggers an attack by the immune system on one's joints, especially the lower vertebrae. The fateful final day in Moscow was the climax of several weeks spent with anxious frustration. The stress hormones required to sustain such anxiety demand that the body cannibalize its reserve of minerals, thus increasing the likelihood of a degenerative bone disease. Cousins was told that in 98.8 percent of cases of rheumatoid spondylitis with a rapid onset of inflammation, the course of the disease is intractable, leading to a severely painful degeneration of the spine.

In 1964, allopathic therapy for rheumatoid spondylitis consisted of bed rest in hospital, twenty-six aspirin and twelve phenylbutazone tablets each day. In consult with his family doctor, Cousins became concerned that chronic use of anti-inflammatories would aggravate a connective tissue disorder. Other aspects of therapy served to convince him that "a hospital is no place for a person who is seriously ill." The food was highly processed, of low nutritional value, and likely to sharply raise blood glucose. He reasoned that being awakened at intervals consistent with hospital schedule does not help any patient, let alone a man recuperating from adrenal exhaustion. At various times in the day he was asked to give blood to each of four distinct hospital departments. I believe Cousins' healing began in earnest when he mustered his energies to post a sign on his door declaring that blood would be given only once every third day.

Fortunately for Cousins, he was able to rent a hotel room across from the hospital where he could be visited by his physicians (of course, by appointment only!). There were many advantages to this arrangement. The room plus a visiting nurse cost only one third as much as a private hospital room. He ordered fresh, low glycemic foods. And, he could freely watch tapes of *Candid Camera* television programs and Marx Brothers movies without his laughter "disturbing" the other patients. His sedimentary rate was found to drop after each viewing, without the use of anti-inflammatory medications. Within a week, the inflammation had dropped in half, and his length of precious, pain-free, undisturbed sleep increased from ten minutes to two hours per night. Over the next six months, Cousins' pain gradually subsided and his mobility returned.

The most significant change in conventional treatment of rheumatoid spondylitis in the past forty years is the implementation of physiotherapy. Daily work with a physical therapist, preferably in a swimming pool, preserves or increases mobility of the spine. There has also been evidence that patients with spondylitis or related rheumatoid diseases suffer from abnormally low levels of vitamin D (25-hydroxy-vitamin-D).[1] Vitamin D is actually a steroid hormone that serves as a natural anti-inflammatory, and helps to regulate the laying down of bone. Studies show the benefits to spondylitis patients, in both their serum vitamin D and pain symptoms, from moderate sun exposure for a three-week period.[2] This is especially appropriate in the dark days of winter and early spring, when diet is insufficient to restore vitamin D levels.

But perhaps the most important factor in successfully managing rheumatoid spondylitis was demonstrated by Cousins' feisty attitude to healing. Patients who tend to play down their symptoms and the stressful nature of their illness are slower to recover. Health care providers need to encourage their patients to assert themselves, which requires listening to their needs and being open to suggestions.

Norman Cousins' *Anatomy of an Illness* should be read, not as a medical protocol, but as testimony to the power of directing one's will to the purpose of healing.[3] On that critical last day in Moscow, Cousins' illness was brought to a head. From here he could have remained "never well since," but his determination to change course was instrumental in relieving his pain, maintaining his spine's integrity, and opening the rest of his life to laughter.

Cousins possessed the political skills to maneuver within the health system. His mental wherewithal to make responsible decisions never flagged because he had a well-tested sense of confidence in the face of authority; his immediate implementation of a plan of action prevented him from falling into a trance-like or depressive state of mind common to patients in hospital.

For most individuals, the longer they persist in a less than healthy state, the harder it becomes to pull themselves free. A protracted illness or a traumatic event increases the likelihood of depression, which, if it persists, will further drain physiologic resources. For example, grief, like the shock following any dramatic intrusion into the course of life, slows us down, makes daily life seem unimportant, and eventually depresses the immune system. A recent meta-analysis found that twenty-eight percent of women newly diagnosed with breast cancer had suffered the loss of a loved one (death, divorce, or separation) within the preceding year.[4] In my own practice, I have seen three cases of breast cancer occurring within months of the death of a loved one. I have also treated three cases of chronic cystitis, two cases of sudden osteoporosis, and a case of multiple sclerosis, each with the same pattern of grief preceding manifestation of disease.

Sometimes, the very tools used to cope with an injury, illness or disease, bind one to a state of poor or mediocre health. For example, taking an anti-depressant might relieve the emotional pain of grief, temporarily making decision-making easier. But, *continued* use of such medications blunts one's emotions and the motivation to engage life issues. Sooner or later, restoration of health will require dealing with the feelings of grief while gradually diminishing reliance on anti-depressants.

Anti-inflammatory drugs are the most commonly prescribed allopathic medications. For example, corticosteroids, used to suppress the body's inflammatory response, effectively reduce unbearable pain, burning or itching sensations; but long-term use reduces the responsiveness of the body's natural anti-inflammatory hormone, cortisol. The longer one uses a synthetic analog such as prednisone or phenylbutazone, the less capable becomes the body to cope on its own. Meanwhile, continued use of corticosteroids will suppress elements of the immune system besides those involved in the inflammatory response, making the patient increasingly vulnerable to infection. In cases such as that of Cousins, the only way to restore health without a growing dependence on anti-inflammatories is to discover and then eliminate as soon as possible the stressor causing the inflammation.

Certain events can damage one's nervous system so as to initiate a chronic illness while simultaneously interfering with the process of decision-making. For example, if the 9-16 week old fetus is exposed to drugs (e.g., alcohol, cocaine), industrial chemicals (e.g., mercury), infectious agents (e.g., cytomegalovirus, varicella virus), or ionizing radiation, then his or her brain will be diminished. Similarly, adults can be exposed to toxic agents or experience a hormonal imbalance that restricts functioning of their central nervous systems.

A perplexing array of evidence for anyone assuming the *influence* paradigm (and the *normative* paradigm to be discussed in Chapter Four) is that even those with extreme neurologic impairment do not necessarily experience a cognitive deficit, emotional impoverishment, or poor decision-making skills. For example, most autopsies performed on the brains of women eighty years of age or older, reveal anatomical evidence of Alzheimer's disease, though only ten percent of these women had exhibited impairment of memory. Without exception, those individuals who had preserved their memory abilities, despite deteriorating memory centers of the brain, had had a history of keeping their minds actively engaged even when suffering with grief or a painful illness.

Frances

The photographs of Frances taken when she was twenty-five years old suggest the rare combination of vigilance and a take-charge personality, the kind of woman you'd want supervising the testing of hazardous chemicals. When I saw her for the first time, she was forty years old, had a glassy-eyed expression, weighed 250 pounds, had not had a menstrual period in three months, awakened feverishly each night, and experienced muscle ache and "heartburn" throughout the day. Like most patients, Frances was looking for remedies to manage each of her symptoms.

An hour into the interview, somewhat embarrassedly Frances revealed that thirteen years earlier she had been diagnosed as schizophrenic, and had been taking anti-psychotic medications ever since. Frances's psychiatrist managed her medications in a diligent and typical manner: find a drug that eliminates symptoms as fast as possible and stay with it until psychiatric symptoms reemerge. For the past five years she has been on risperidone. As is the case with most psychiatric medications, risperidone has been tested only in short-term trials (six-eight weeks). Though it is considered "therapy," long-term use of such medications is, in fact, part of an ongoing test of the drug's efficacy and safety.

In test patients it was not uncommon for resperidone to induce (within six to eight weeks) increased sleepiness, indigestion, muscle pain, changes in muscle tone, fever, anxiety with heart palpitations, or irregular menses; and obesity is a common outcome of any long-term anti-psychotic therapy. Since all of Frances's presenting symptoms appear to be the side-effect of managing her schizophrenia, I asked her what were the symptoms that had led to her diagnosis. She did not recall any of her doctors, since her first psychiatric evaluation, inquiring into the circumstances leading to her diagnosis.

Frances had been the laboratory technician supervising the study of a new chemical amalgam that included methyl bromide, chlorine, xylene, toluene, cyanate, arsenic, cadmium, and acetone. Under pressure, the compound "went aerosol," poisoning her assistant and herself. They both spent two days in intensive care and another day under hospital observation before being released. While her assistant recovered with no signs of neurologic damage, Frances was found the following day staggering down the middle of a busy highway. The company doctor of course recognized the cause of her psychotic behavior as being due to the chemical spill, and authorized her disability reimbursement, along with a prescription for anti-psychotic medication.

Unfortunately, two years later Frances still was unable to work, with diminished short-term memory and stretches of time when she appeared disoriented (not being able to communicate the day of the week or her own whereabouts). The subsequent psychiatric interview found that she had never experienced a psychotic break with reality before the accident. This in itself should be a red flag to a psychologist or psychiatrist bent on a diagnosis: non-toxic cases of schizophrenia almost always appear gradually over time. However, the psychiatrist noted that the assistant had been exposed to the same chemicals but had fully recovered, and therefore concluded that Frances probably had had a *latent* psychosis triggered by the spill. Such gamesmanship with words seems to be necessary in order to hold onto the *normative* paradigm. Instead of looking at the evidence for individual differences in response to environmental toxins, the psychiatrist asserted the existence of a psychosis that no one could have detected.

Each of the chemicals to which Frances had been exposed has been documented in the medical literature as being neurotoxic. For example, over 400 cases of methyl bromide poisoning have been shown to cause convulsions, an unstable gait, loss of short-term memory, decreased vocabulary, or confused speech. The ability of the liver to detoxify and excrete such chemicals varies greatly between people, with some individuals clearing drugs up to forty-five times faster than others. For example, the British journal *Occupational Medicine* reported an incident of two experienced fumigation workers simultaneously exposed to methyl bromide, only one of whom retained high blood levels of the poison, causing him to remain bedridden for five months.[5]

The liver and small intestine have responsibility for detoxification. Potentially toxic chemicals are not only ingested as components of drugs, but also consumed on a daily basis in food and water, and absorbed through the skin. Even the healthiest foods yield toxic by-products in the normal process of digestion. For example, ammonia produced by bacteria as they metabolize amino acids is converted by liver enzymes into the less toxic urea molecule. If, however, the liver fails to make this conversion, ammonia intoxication will cause central nervous system damage that produces tremors, slurred speech and eventually coma and death. Those with poor liver detoxification should be cautious about dramatically reducing their protein and sugar intake. In the first week of a fast, large amounts of ammonia are dumped into the blood stream as the body catabolizes its muscle tissue for the necessary amino acids.

Steroid hormones and most drugs pose a danger since they are fat-soluble, while excretion from the body depends upon a chemical being mixed with water-based fluids such as urine, sweat, or conjugated bilirubin (a constituent of feces). The liver makes fat-soluble chemicals water-soluble, using one or both of the following detoxification pathways. So-called *oxidative* reactions use the enzyme cytochrome p450 to add an oxygen atom to the molecule. A second, *conjugation*, reaction binds the toxin to a water-soluble molecule (glycine, glucuronic acid, or a sulphur molecule). The most lipophilic (Greek, *fat loving*) chemicals require first the addition of oxygen and then binding to a water-soluble molecule, while moderately lipophilic chemicals are detoxified by conjugation alone.

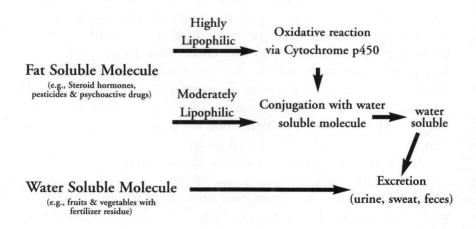

Figure 3.1. Detoxification pathways.

The consequence of having complex and multiple biochemical pathways is that our bodies have mechanisms and backup systems to accommodate the choices we make. For example, most people taking fat-soluble drugs soon begin to gain a girth of fat cells. Detoxification pathways have their limits, beyond which drug metabolites are stored away from the blood system in fat cells. So important is this sequestration into fat reserves that we find multiple pathways to accomplish it. For example, anti-psychotic drugs raise levels of blood glucose, triglycerides, and adrenal steroid hormones, as well as neurotransmitters that increase appetite; all of this leads to the creation and continued maintenance of extra fat cells.

Frances is among the majority of patients taking anti-psychotic drugs who have consequently become obese. Besides the drug metabolites being stored within her fat cells, there are almost certainly chemical remnants of the initial toxic spill. Whenever she had attempted to lose weight, she had felt flu-like symptoms (including nausea, headaches and muscle aches) indicative of dumping of toxins from fat cells into the blood stream. In such cases, it is essential to have the detoxification pathways working at maximum efficiency before initiating the burning of fat. In Frances' case, this was desirable because (a) her obesity was a threat to her cardiovascular health, (b) the drug metabolites were placing an ever-increasing burden on the detoxification pathways, and (c) toxic spill remnants might be slowly leaking into her blood system.

The oxidative detoxification pathway produces free radicals that can damage the nervous system. Therefore, we had Frances begin supplementing her diet with a natural form of vitamin E (400 IU three times per day); in conjunction with vitamin C (500 mg twice daily) and selenium (200 mcg at bedtime) her body would then have the building blocks for the antioxidant glutathione. Vitamin E, the oil of rosemary, and the hormones melatonin and DHEA have each been found to protect the nervous system from peroxidation of fats and detoxification by-products. She still enjoys sprinkling rosemary oil on bread, vegetables and salad. I recommended DHEA (50 mg) rather than melatonin because Frances had symptoms of hormonal imbalance. We also created a multi-vitamin/

mineral including good amounts of the B vitamins, and the minerals molybdenum and zinc.

The conjugation pathway depends upon the amino acid glycine, the glucose-derived molecule glucuronic acid, and nutrients that provide sulphur. Foods that contain or promote these nutrients include eggs, wheat germ, elderberries, brazil nuts, muscles, oysters, octopus, canned "light" tuna, artichokes, cooked cauliflower, and the spice turmeric. I cautioned Frances to avoid alcohol, caffeine, pork, beef, aged cheese, or MSG (often hidden with the label "flavorings"), as each of these puts an extra burden on the detoxification pathways, and to some extent competes with the beneficial nutrients.

With some encouragement, Frances made an appointment to see her psychiatrist, and requested that he lower the dose of her medications. Physicians are reluctant to reduce or change medications when there are no new negative side effects. However, when patients point out the problems they are experiencing (in this case obesity, muscle pain, and amenorrhea) and step forward to take responsibility for the consequences of a change in medication, physicians will generally change their drug regimen. Frances's psychiatrist suggested reducing her risperidone by half.

We were now ready to begin burning fat and expurgating toxins. In the absence of fatty or sugary foods, the body will scream pangs of hunger for three or four days before burning its fat stores for energy. For the first three days of the "fast" Frances ate unlimited quantities of steamed vegetables: artichokes, cauliflower, kale, carrots, green beans, mustard greens, and butternut squash. These could be spiced with turmeric, garlic, onion or red pepper. She took a dropper-full of ginger bitters before each meal to stimulate digestion. Each day she drank two quarts of lemon juice or wheat grass juice, and two quarts of low-particulate water (less than five parts per million). Besides the above-mentioned vitamins, minerals and DHEA, Frances took four grams of glycine powder (about one level teaspoon) mixed with her juice. For days four through six, she added to her menu yams, apples, cherries, apricots, and elderberries. On each of the subsequent days, she introduced into her diet a different food: soft-boiled eggs, whole wheat cereal, brazil nuts, and lastly crustaceans and "light" tuna.

The systematic reintroduction of foods serves the additional function of detecting a food allergy. It takes approximately five days for immune antigens to clear out of the blood system after one's last encounter with an allergy-provoking molecule. When the offender is reintroduced, allergic symptoms become quite noticeable. In Frances's case, her nasal sinuses congested when she reintroduced the wheat cereal, and cleared after eliminating wheat from her diet.

To facilitate fat burning, Frances started an exercise program. The energy required for the initial minutes of any exercise is drawn from available carbohydrates. When the carbohydrates are used up, the exerciser feels tired or "winded" or "hits the wall." Frances encountered the "fat wall" after only three or four minutes of vigorous walking since she was in poor condition to begin with, and she was eating a low carbohydrate diet. The temptation is to then stop and rest, but if one perseveres through this period, the body will start to metabolize fat rather than sugar, and the exerciser will experience a "second wind."

After shifting to fat metabolization, people with "fat to burn" can continue comfortably exercising until oxygen levels fail to keep pace with demand (causing a sharp rise in lactic acid in the muscles). The length of time prior to feeling the lactic acid burn can be maximized by efficient oxygen use. Based on studies of athletes in training, I suggested to Frances that she breathe in and out through her nose, and to continue walking a brisk pace until she felt compelled to breathe through her mouth. The body will resist going into oxygen debt by reflexively accessing a larger channel of air, namely by opening the mouth. I instructed her to continue walking when this happened, but to slow down to the point where she could breathe normally again.

After three days, Frances was able to walk briskly for thirty minutes without stopping. This facilitated the release of toxins from her fat cells, as well as the elimination of toxins from her body. Aerobic exercise provides an outlet for toxins through the breath as well as the skin, and decreases bowel transit time.

Meanwhile, a whole-foods diet with increased fluid intake generally makes the stools softer and the bowels more regular, thus improving elimination of waste material.

After ten days, Frances felt greater overall vitality, though her hands ached more than usual. She began to sense a familiar smell or taste of bromide, which made her memory of the events surrounding the chemical spill clearer. In fact, sitting five or six feet away, I could detect a chemical aroma coming from her body. The increased achiness and the chemical smell or taste indicated that she had liberated toxins into her blood stream. To facilitate detoxification, we added 500 mg glucuronic acid to her daily regimen, and three minutes of sauna every other day. When using a sauna for detoxification, it is important to towel off *before* taking a warm shower. This extends the time skin pores stay clear and capable of excreting toxic-filled sweat.

At the end of week five, Frances had lost thirteen pounds, was continuing to feel greater energy, had no muscle discomfort, had lost the chemical taste and smell, and experienced her first menstrual period in five months. For the first time, she looked and sounded emotionally expressive. Her face and tone of voice appeared animated.

She confided to me that she had heard voices counseling her every move during the past fifteen years. Her anti-psychotic medications had made it easier to discount the voices, but the voices had never gone away until this week. I took this opportunity to ask Frances about the nature of the hallucinations.

"Tell me about the voices you heard; for example, how did they sound?"

After some reflection, she answered, "The tone of the voice was like the voice you hear in your head when thinking."

"Is that voice male or female, young or old?"

"It was *my* tone of voice, but spoken by someone else."

I asked, "Can you say how many different speakers there were? And could you still hear your own voice?"

"I didn't think about it, but I guess there were three or four speakers. When I wasn't too tired, I'd *shout* in my mind to keep things straight. When I got tired, I'd just listen to the others."

I sensed that Frances was apprehensive that the voices might return unless she remained vigilant. I communicated my confidence that her dissociative symptoms were finished. "Suppose you take a deep breath, right now, and relax it out. Just let your mind wander to whatever…Perhaps you'll feel the air from your breath on your upper lip, or your eyes relaxing closed…The mind is wonderful in that it can think of just about anything and then return when ready…"

After a minute, Frances opened her eyes, smiled and commented that she hadn't heard anything. I asked, "Do you ever think, but not in words?"

A moment later, her eyes teared. "I love music." Her eyes closed, her left foot began tapping, and Frances appeared content. It was the first time in recent years that she had allowed herself to mentally recreate and then enjoy a tune that she had listened to before the accident. From where I sat, I could just hear a little humming.

Doctor Shiva

I saw Doctor Shiva for little more than one session. He was a young surgeon unable to stop his hands from shaking.

During his general internship, he began suffering from migraine headaches. Because he served at a large American teaching hospital, he was asked to undergo a spinal tap to rule out infectious meningitis and to serve as an example of the procedure. This procedure would certainly not have been performed had he been a typical patient since there is the potential for complications and meningitis is not a very likely cause. In fact, migraines are common for those working through the stress of becoming a physician.

Unfortunately, Shiva's procedure went awry. A puncture causing spinal fluid to leak when standing required him to remain in bed for the next six months. Subsequently, he had managed the headaches and tremors allopathically by taking ever-increasing amounts of sedatives. But, at some point, a sedated surgeon is no more effective than a shaking one.

Now, five years after starting his practice, his MRI was normal though his symptoms had become unmanageable. I pointed out that his symptoms had grown worse the more medications he had ingested. It made sense to Dr. Shiva that we had no notion of what underlying condition we might be dealing with while he was taking a potpourri of drugs. He must have been desperate because he agreed to stop working for a week and also to go off all medications. Meanwhile, he followed a liver detoxification diet consisting of cooked vegetables and vegetable juices. To facilitate detoxification and buffer the withdrawal from sedatives, he took a teaspoon of the amino acid glycine in juice throughout the day.

One week later, Shiva walked into my office, put out both hands steady as a rock, and walked out without a word.

Jackie

In the glory days of allopathic medicine that followed World War II, a physician was respected by his peers for his ability to accurately and rapidly diagnose a patient's injury or disease. Once a patient had been assigned to a diagnostic category, the best treatment known to help the largest number of patients with that condition would then be applied. This methodology has been complicated in the past thirty years by an ever-increasing number of "syndromes" with which a physician may categorize a patient. Syndromes, unlike diseases, are collections of signs and symptoms known to arise from any number of possible causes. The proliferation of syndrome categories reflects a deepening understanding of physiology and biochemistry and how those pathways uniquely intertwine in response to the patient. Consequently, today's most successful physicians enjoy the role of detective perhaps even more than being a repository of medical information.

Jackie had suffered with chronic fatigue syndrome (CFS) for four years. She mustered up enough energy to get to my office and collapse into the chair across from me. Fifty years old, five-foot-seven and 105 pounds, she looked gaunt and haggard. She was understandably depressed by her memory of having been physically vital. Jackie had loved being a kindergarten teacher and competitive tennis player. She had been "going down hill" since having a urinary tract infection. Now, the least physical exertion would cause physical and mental incapacitation, effectively preventing her from engaging in any work or play.

CFS involves a spiraling drain of energy that could be initiated by any stressful event. Inevitably, it is caused by a combination of stressors that progressively tax every physiological and psychological system. The most severe cases begin with an infection or exposure to toxins either of which activates an inflammatory response by the immune system. The resulting chemicals serve to fight the infection

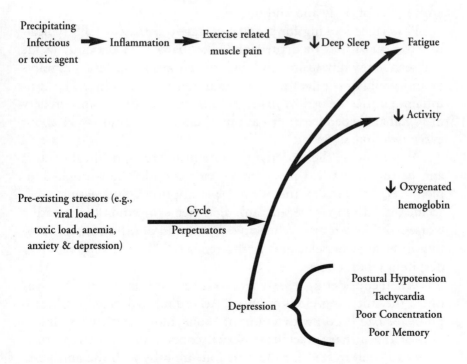

Figure 3.2. Initiation and perpetuation of severe chronic fatigue syndrome.

or expel toxins, but also increase exercise-related muscle pain and cause the central nervous system to decrease time in deep sleep. A consequence is fatigue and a need to decrease physical activity. Reduced exercise means the brain receives less oxygenated hemoglobin, which eventually causes postural hypotension (falling blood pressure after standing up), tachycardia (racing heart beat), and poor concentration and short-term memory. In turn, these symptoms make one feel depressed, with even less desire to be active.

The course that CFS takes differs from that of a common infection or toxic exposure in that there are additional aggravating circumstances that perpetuate the vicious cycle. For example, the flu by itself commonly causes fatigue and even some depression, but will, within days or weeks, be resolved. However, if there is also a long history of viral infections or anemia an acute illness may turn chronic, and thereby engender a deepening depression and a progressive atrophying of body and endurance.

Physicians looking for a single causative entity for CFS typically settle on viruses or depression. Like many CFS patients, Jackie had seen many physicians, and undertaken various generic programs of anti-viral, anti-inflammatory, and mood altering drugs. The anti-inflammatories helped to manage pain symptoms; the anti-anxiety drug Xanax helped her to fall asleep, though she would awake about every two hours.

Not knowing the underlying cause of *her* CFS, medical doctors and chiropractors had plied Jackie with countless nutritional supplements. In spite of the various prescriptions, and eating what seemed a "healthy" (vegetarian) diet, her symptoms had steadily worsened. No diet or psychoactive drug could diminish Jackie's profound sense of hopelessness as she reflected, "Life is slipping away despite my best efforts."

When considering a *never well since* case, it is imperative to scrutinize the initiating circumstances. According to Jackie, her health problems had begun with a bout of "honeymoon cystitis," an infection of the urinary tract from sexual contact with a new partner. This had been treated for the next four months with the antibiotic Bactrim, when she suddenly experienced nausea, a pounding occipital headache, and overall weakness. Her HMO medical doctor, believing the bladder infection to be resolved and facing a collection of symptoms that does not fit neatly into a disease category, reasoned that the problem must be psychiatric rather than medical. He accordingly diagnosed Jackie as having panic attacks, prescribed Xanax, and referred her to a psychiatrist.

Often there is a matrix of precipitating events that have been organized in the patient's mind under one temporal landmark ("the bladder infection"). By having Jackie explicate those events, she revealed that soon after the honeymoon cystitis, her boyfriend "walked out on her." The pain around her menses dramatically increased, and a year later she was diagnosed with uterine cancer that was surgically removed with a hysterectomy.

The patient's narrative provides a wealth of symptoms: different "streams of consciousness" that connect the past, present and future, and hidden clues we gather en route to an explanation that points the way to a cure. Detective work in a complex case requires a combination of careful observation, digging up of evidence, and time to allow the various hypotheses to" incubate." As in any creative endeavor, the incubation stage allows ideas to develop as one looks at the whole picture from multiple perspectives.

Jackie brought in the results of a stool sample and the record of her complete blood counts and urinalyses. Her blood tests showed no consistent pattern of pathology, but the urine and stool samples showed her to be abnormally alkaline (high pH). This I confirmed by having her place pH paper in her mouth: it turned a dark green color, indicating a high level of alkalinity.

During our first consultation, I took notes listing her many symptoms, objective measures (e.g., pH), and my assessment of possible causes. These notes have been cleaned up and presented in Figure 3.3.

Reflecting on my notes, it was apparent that, from the perspective of Ayurvedic medicine, many of her symptoms should be grouped together as a disturbance in *Vata*: weight loss from poor digestion, cold and dry skin, easily fatigued from exertion, and a body and mind that react to changes in the environment. In gener-

CC (Chief Complaint)
>   Fatigue, pain on exertion, poor memory,
>   1998: positive for multiple viruses (including EBV).
>   1998 (M.D.) diagnosis of Chronic Fatigue Syndrome.

S (Subjective)
>   Little sensation in hands & feet.
>   Muscle & joint pain persists for days after minimal exercise.
>   Gas after eating.
>   Primarily raw vegetable diet.
>   Chronic constipation.
>   Feels depressed thinking about her limitations.
>   Feels "scared and out of control."
>   "Takes on others' stuff" (distress).
>   "Xanax takes edge off symptoms & helps sleep."
>   NWS boyfriend walking out—-Recurrent UTI—-antibiotics.

O (Objective)
>   105 lbs, 5'7"
>   Pale, cold, dry skin.
>   Pulses: Kidney Yang is "frantic," Kidney Yin not palpable.
>   BP: 105/65 (standing), 90/60 (sitting), reactive.
>   Elevated pH: stool (7.8), urine, saliva.

A (Assessment)
>   Vata disturbance.
>   Postural hypotension.
>   Refractory depression.
>   Hypoacidic.

P (Plan)
>   Ginger, Panax, licorice tincture, tid.
>   "Ginger Bitters" before meals.
>   Low-glycemic diet.
>   Rebalance pH with diet.
>   Seafood, tofu, currants, eggs, yoghurt, black tea, steamed vegetables,
>   hemp oil.
>   Colostrum.
>   Gradually increase exercise; gentle walk in sunlight.
>   Lycopodium 200C in office.

Figure 3.3. Abridged case notes from Jackie's first consultation.

al, the Ayurvedic prescription for a *Vata* disorder is to (a) increase digestive "fire", (b) increase the availability of fluids to the various connective tissues, (c) provide a nutritious diet, and (d) begin a regular program of gentle exercise.

I prescribed an herbal formula in the form of a tincture added to her black tea, with the intention of serving both Ayurvedic and Western allopathic medicine. The remedy contained ginger which is warming and stimulates digestion; Panax ginseng which is warming, supports adrenal function, increases stamina, and stimulates interferon production; and licorice which moistens, raises blood pressure, stimulates interferon production and is anti-inflammatory.

I recommended that she adjust her diet so as to increase her intake of protein and fat, and to establish an acid-alkaline balance. The common foods listed in Figure 3.4 have not been organized by their chemical composition, but rather by their affect on blood pH. My recommendations took into account the need to protect the immune system, diminish the incidence of lactic acid "burn," while not taxing her digestive system. Accordingly, I encouraged Jackie to avoid both alkaline and extremely acid-forming foods while focusing on eating figs, currants, plums, guava, string beans, chard, tofu, brown rice, wheat, Jerusalem artichokes, clarified butter, yogurt, and black tea. Since she had chosen to "give up meat for health rather than philosophy," I recommended that she reintroduce into her diet eggs, fish, shrimp and lamb.

Implementing a regular program of exercise in a graduated manner can pose a challenge. Most CFS patients learn to not trust their bodies and are, therefore, reluctant to engage in any exercise. But, for people like Jackie, who remember long, invigorating hours playing at sports, the tendency is to over tax one's energy reserves when feeling some vitality. Fortunately, she agreed to *gradually* increase her activity level, initially by walking to her backyard in the late morning. I encouraged her to wait a few days before walking down the block to a park bench.

I did not see Jackie for the next eighteen months, during which time she "hit the circuit" of CFS specialists. She looked like an emaciated boxer.

Highly Acidifying	Moderately Acidifying	Moderately Alkalizing	Highly Alkalizing
sugar, aspartame	honey, maple syrup	Sucanat	mineral water
white vinegar	basalmic vinegar	apple cider vinegar	sea vegetables
cocoa, carob	sulphured molasses	unsulphured molasses	
ice cream			
alcohol, coffee, cola	Kona coffee, black tea	green tea, sake	
walnuts, brazils, pecans, pistachios,		almonds, chestnuts	pumpkin seeds poppy seeds
walnut oil	canola, almond, sesame, grapeseed, pumpkin, & corn oils	coconut & olive oils	
nutmeg	vanilla, iodized salt	most herbs	sea salt, garlic, cinnamon
barley, corn, rye	wheat, rice	oats, wild rice, quinoa	
soy beans, peanuts	beans, spinach, miso, peas, tofu	squash, eggplant, potato lettuce, cauliflower mushrooms, peppers	lentils, onion, root vegetables kale, broccoli
cranberries pomegranate	tomato, plum, guava dried fruit	apple, berries, peach, pear papaya, cherry orange apricot, banana, kiwi, grapes, avocado	melons, lemon, lime, grapefruit, mango, nectarine, persimmon, pineapple
beef, pork, lobster, chicken	fish, game, lamb, crustaceans, duck, eggs		
soft cheese, processed cheese	aged cheese, milk,	cultured milk	

Figure 3.4. The Effect of Food on Body pH

"So, was it the diet that drove you away?"

Jackie got the joke and answered slowly, "I spoke with a nutritionist who said I should eat alkaline foods and stay vegetarian, so I didn't know what to do".

"Are you feeling better?"

She raised her eyebrows, "Not really; I could barely get myself here today".

On two occasions, specialists had given her a series of anti-viral drugs that had precipitated a complete collapse. The last specialist had provided Jackie with a complete blood count that included a measurement that caught my attention. Her mean cell volume (MCV) was an abnormally high 104, indicating megaloblastic anemia. A red blood cell will grow in volume when cell division cannot keep up with cell growth. The DNA pathway that determines cell division requires vitamins B12 and folate. When these coenzymes are not available in sufficient quantities, red blood cells grow large and are destroyed faster than they can be produced. The resulting anemia causes tissues to receive insufficient amounts of oxygen. This affects the cardiovascular system by making the individual short of breath after relatively little exertion. It affects the central nervous system, predisposing one to headaches and dizziness. Vitamins B12 and folate are also essential to chemical pathways that maintain healthy nerve cells.

Because of their interdependence, vitamin B12 insufficiency (pernicious anemia) or folic acid anemia can lead to the same fatigue and neurologic symptoms. If the problem is a diet lacking folate-rich leafy greens or animal products rich in B12, pathologic symptoms will manifest after several years, as the body's stores are slowly used up. However, if the vitamin stores are destroyed by drugs or chemical by-products, symptoms may begin after only a few days.

We were now in a position to understand from a biochemical point of view how Jackie's CFS had begun. Bactrim kills bacteria by interfering with the folic acid pathways with which they need to grow. By the same mechanism, the antibiotic caused folic acid anemia in Jackie, with symptoms appearing as her body ran out of folate.

Enlarged red blood cells did not manifest for years, not until she also depleted her stores of vitamin B12. The pernicious anemia undoubtedly came about from a combination of factors: (a) increased demand for B12 to compensate for the loss of folate, (b) a primarily vegetarian diet, lacking B12, and (c) diminished ability to absorb B12. Vitamin B12 absorption is dependent upon the stomach secreting sufficient amounts of hydrochloric acid in order to extract the vitamin from typically protein-rich foods. Jackie is highly alkaline, implying an insufficient amount of protein-digesting acid. At least as important is the fact that in order to manage pain, Jackie had taken NSAIDs (non-steroidal anti-inflammatory drugs) on a regular basis for the past seven years. The stomach puts out a molecule called *intrinsic factor* that binds with B12, making it available for assimilation. Prolonged use of almost any NSAID depletes intrinsic factor and predisposes one to a bleeding, anemia-aggravating leaky gut (a condition where toxic matter or undigested food leaks from the bowels into the blood stream).

Jackie learned to give herself intramuscular injections of vitamin B12 (1000 mcg every other day for a month), and took folic acid tablets (800 mcg) each morning and afternoon. In place of the herbal tincture, she enjoyed a teaspoon of licorice solid extract each morning. She agreed to stop taking ibuprofen, and began implementing an acidifying diet.

After two months of treatment, Jackie's energy was obviously returning and she had gained a few pounds. She braved a declaration that anyone with a chronic illness is reluctant to make: "I think I am getting better." She was taking classes in ballroom dancing and colored her hair to look more attractive.

Jackie repeatedly postponed follow-up visits to my office, ostensibly for financial reasons. When I next saw her, a year had passed. Though her skin had a healthy color and she had obviously put on muscle, Jackie still had muscle pain in her legs that prevented her from resuming teaching. She was reading the various internet sites on *fibromyalgia*, and taking nutritional supplements sold by a local chiropractor.

Whenever dealing with chronic illness it is valuable to inquire whether patients are getting something from their illness that might be deterring them from making healthy choices. I decided to probe Jackie about her "perfectly healthy life prior to the bladder infection." After some discussion, Jackie revealed that when she was five years old, her father had walked out on the family; she had fallen ill, and was made to feel thoroughly loved by her mother. In fact, thereafter, she has felt loved *only* when sick.

Seven years ago, she had felt "shocked and amazed" when her lover had abandoned her, leaving behind "only his germs." Her "sickness gives you love" schema did not create her boyfriend's urinary tract bacteria and viruses, or even the subsequent reaction to Bactrim, but it might have been helping to *maintain* the CFS and the "fibromyalgia."

Whenever dealing with chronic illness it is valuable to inquire whether patients are getting something from their illness that might be deterring them from making healthy choices.

After further discussion, Jackie recognized herself in the Type C personality: (a) manifesting cancer within a year of breaking up with her boyfriend, (b) mentally associating sickness and love, (c) taking on guilt for her father's abandonment, (d) subjugating her needs to those of others. Jackie admitted that when feeling a return of vitality, she had also felt guilty because she was "feeling better and others aren't."

I posed the question to Jackie as to how she might put this insight to good use. She soon reflected that her mother was also someone who dealt with other's needs before her own, though she had always been "strong and capable."

"I assume that your mother was strong when your father left, and capable of taking care of you and your house by herself?"

"Of course, though I don't think she ever loved another man."

"And, of course, that is not something you could ever give her. But you are stronger now, so maybe…"

"It's time for me to visit mom. She's alone and could use a hand refurbishing the old house."

David

Homo sapiens have an unsurpassed ability to adapt to life-threatening circumstances. The dilemma facing each of us is that, while adaptation is necessary for survival, most change involves discomfort. With increasing distance from the precipitating event, we lose memory of what we have suffered, but we also find ourselves floating down a stream without knowing where we began or the choices we have made. Illness can awaken one to this unsettling state of affairs. As the fog begins to lift we may discern that all about us is fertile soil to nurture our decisions into anything from genius to disability.

David and I have been friends ever since medical school. At twenty-five years of age, he was one of the younger students. He was muscular, athletic, with a quick mind and an infectious laugh that bordered on a cackle. Two years earlier he had found his biological mother as part of a growing interest in self-discovery. In this spirit, he asked me to work up his *homeopathic constitution*.

Homeopathy is a school of medicine originating with Samuel Hahnemann in the nineteenth century, with its roots in the theory and practice of Hippocrates. The goal of the homeopathic physician is to support and stimulate the body-mind complex to heal itself. A constitutional portrait takes into account every aspect of the person, and constitutional remedies serve to wake up and concentrate the body's ability to organize itself. As such, I began to assemble a picture of David's health history as well as present symptomology.

David had suffered throughout his life with muscle spasms affecting his throat, neck, back, and bladder. His neck (cervical) muscles would often become painfully rigid. He would suddenly get a "lump in the throat" from muscle spasms about the larynx. His reflexes were hyper-responsive and his consciousness hypervigilant to events in his environment. He tended to be restless, unable to sit for more than a few minutes at a time. Ever since being a young child David had been treated for epilepsy. In fact, some of his most pleasant memories were of grand mal seizures: "perfectly alert, calm and unable to move."

I checked the homeopathic repertories for these symptoms and found that, as a whole, they were similar to symptoms that arise from strychnine poisoning. Homeopathic investigators were the first scientists to use double blind, placebo-controlled methodology. Subjects given dilute quantities of strychnine or juice expressed from plants containing strychnine (e.g. *Ignatia*, or *Nux vomica*) rapidly developed acute symptoms of muscle spasms in back, larynx or bladder, grand mal seizures, as well as hyper-responsiveness and mental hyperacuity.

David had no knowledge of his being exposed to strychnine, and so we considered events that might have occurred when he was too young to remember. His biological mother recalled that it was a difficult birth that led to the injection of a muscle relaxant to induce labor. Tubocurarine was the neuromuscular block consistently used for this purpose. The only potential complication of this procedure is that if labor is not forthcoming in ten minutes, the drug enters the blood circulation of the infant. David's mother recalls the panic in the hospital staff when she failed to dilate sufficiently and delivery was delayed for another hour (instead of the recommended cesarean section). Tubocurarine is an extract of curare, the strychnine-rich poison traditionally used by South American Indians to stun their prey.

After making such a connection in the patient's history, a homeopathic practitioner will consider giving the patient a highly dilute derivative of the precipitating poison. The goal would be to direct the body's attention to those symptoms associated with strychnine poisoning, though, this time, without suffering a toxic dose of the drug.

It happens that none of the common strychnine homeopathic remedies are associated with a mental picture that looks much like David. *Nux vomica* was the closest in that it has helped those with grand mal seizures: the homeopathic *Materia Medica* includes,

"Very clear consciousness while unable to respond." However, a constitutional remedy should represent not just pathological symptoms, but also the person at his or her healthiest. *Nux vomica* typically helps the workaholic who self-medicates to get through the day. This simply did not fit David's personality, and so we continued to explore his earliest memories. (Today, I probably would have prescribed *Nux vomica* as a first remedy. Because I was not yet a physician, I was not expected to automatically know the answer, and was therefore afforded time to incubate and research the problem.)

I asked David about the earliest dream he could remember. He vividly recalled a recurrent dream of being tied down and pierced through the chest with arrows. This "dream" is probably related to an early experience accompanying a seizure. I hunted for this dream image in the homeopathic literature. Out of the thousands of substances that have been studied homeopathically, I was excited to discover that, "Dreams of being pierced through chest with arrows" is elicited in response to one substance: *Bombyx processiana,* the caterpillar in cocoon. We find in the *Chinese Materia Medica* that *Bombyx* has one specific use: "inhibits, in young children, seizures/convulsions caused by strychnine."[6]

David and I were elated at this revelation. He calmly telephoned his father and asked him to tell me about David's great hobby as a child. He had enjoyed collecting caterpillars and watching them become Monarch butterflies! He hated the idea of pinning them into a scrapbook, but rather loved setting them free.

Within two weeks we had obtained a homeopathic dilution of *Bombyx.* After two doses, David was more relaxed physically and mentally; he appeared centered and more mature. That weekend, David met "the woman of my dreams" and was married a few months later.

It would be a mistake to conclude that the homeopathic remedy determined David's life any more than did his fetal toxicity. The process of healing began with David's search for his roots; homeopathic *Bombyx* and the discovery of what it represents helped to make sense of events in his life, naturally allowing him to set himself free.

Every fetus that develops into infancy has had to adapt to chemical and structural interference, including everything from a strawberry daiquiri to a bumpy motor scooter ride. For the most part, these adaptations fall within what society considers "normal variability" and are, therefore, not noticed. Other children adapting to fetal stress may look normal, though, like David, they develop divergent reactions and behaviors.

A problem for anyone subscribing to the influence paradigm is that individuals with the same degree of pathology may choose to pursue very different lives. For any pathologic condition with an obvious beginning, and where the individual can make responsible decisions, there is a choice of acting on one's life as either "never well since" or "challenged ever since." In such cases, our role as physicians can only be to remind patients that they have the power to navigate their own lives, and to assist them in what is often a heroic effort.

Telemachus

Temporal landmarks punctuate the narrative of one's life with meaning. Some of these events are intensely personal, other events are shared with certain individuals, and still others exist as part of the collective story of one's society. Unfortunately, having an event to mark the beginnings of an illness may keep one close to that illness since it provides light in an otherwise dark and lonely passage.

Telly was diagnosed with Crohn's disease (CD) three years ago, when he was thirty-two years of age. CD is a chronic inflammation of the intestines that causes severe abdominal pain, diarrhea, nausea, and weight loss. Telly sees this as the most recent in a line of illnesses stretching back to his being sexually abused at the age of nine by older boys.

Silently, he lived with fear of being gang-raped. For Telly, there was, and still is, shame attached to his sense of powerlessness. We had several sessions before Telly shared with me that this horror had continued for almost five years. With puberty, Telly decided to develop his body: "No more ninety-pound weakling for me." In fact, he worked at becoming athletic so diligently, that by twenty he was a world-class cross-country bicycle racer.

Working with athletes poses special problems to the health care practitioner. Athletes, unlike most of us, take "coaching" very seriously, and, given that their goal is to push beyond normal limits, take recommendations to their extreme. For example, upon hearing

---

It is best to direct the athlete's attention to the sensation of balance, and the distinction between the soreness of expanding one's limits and the pain from pushing too fast.

---

of the virtues of fish oil, an athlete like Telly will stock his larder with sardines, eat fresh fish for lunch and dinner, and take Omega-3 capsules for breakfast! They also have learned to associate pain with progress in their training ("No pain, no gain"). On the other hand, athletes are wonderfully sensitive to the needs of their bodies, and signs that their bodies are out of balance. For these reasons, it is best to direct the athlete's attention to the sensation of balance, and the distinction between the soreness of expanding one's limits and the pain from pushing too fast. They typically respond to the challenge of maintaining a dynamic balance that allows them to expand without the danger of injury. With this as their goal, athletes can determine for themselves exactly how much or how little is enough.

At nineteen, Telly was in a bicycle accident that caused a deep bruise to his right kidney. He had bloody urine on and off for the next three years but pushed forward with his competitions. At twenty-two, Telly experienced an emotionally charged event that appears to have interacted with the compromised state of his kidney. Following a heated argument, his girlfriend called the police and had him removed from their home. Having his neighbors see him in handcuffs was mortifying. He became profoundly depressed, and three months later was diagnosed with nephrotic syndrome, an imbalance in kidney function in which water is held in the tissues and protein is expelled through the urine.

As with any syndrome, nephrotic syndrome can arise from many potential causes, or, more often, a combination of precipitating events. At a physiologic level, it is caused either by white blood cells damaging the kidney, or as part of a disease (e.g., diabetes, lupus, cancer, infections, or drug reactions) that affects various body systems. The recommended allopathic therapy is very different for the two etiologies, necessitating an accurate assessment prior to prescribing a drug. For example, it can be life threatening to suppress the immune system in a patient who is actually suffering from diabetes, cancer, or an infection.

Telly's physician saw no signs of a systemic disease and therefore put him on prednisone and cyclosporine in order to suppress any immune reaction. Signs and symptoms of nephritis receded, but within a year the cyclosporine had caused Telly's hair to fall out, and the prednisone had elevated his blood sugar and pushed him into insulin dependent diabetes.

By the time I first saw Telly, eleven years later, he had had numerous acute episodes associated with nephrotic syndrome, had an early stage of macular degeneration (loss of central retinal cells) from poorly controlled blood sugar, and was suffering from painful symptoms of Crohn's disease. The number of prescription medications had, of course, kept pace with the number of illnesses, with increasing doses of cyclosporine and prednisone, and periodic series of antibiotics.

Corticosteroids such as prednisone relieve inflammatory signs and symptoms of CD, but also power a vicious cycle of progressive drug dependence and destruction of the intestines. A suppressed immune system makes the intestines more vulnerable to bacteria, which, in turn, elicits an inflammatory response. Throwing antibiotics into the mix will kill most bacteria, but eventually promotes resistant-strains while killing off beneficial bacteria. Furthermore, the intestines will often adapt to suppressive steroids by laying down granular sheets of white blood cells (*malacoplakia*). The resulting inflammation is typically treated with higher doses of steroids or NSAIDs (e.g., Tylenol) until the intestine perforates and requires surgical resectioning.

In order to exit the spiraling cycle of drugs and inflammation, we decided to manage Telly's inflammation without steroids and without anti-inflammatories that erode the lining of the digestive system. He began taking a classic collection of herbal extracts known as Robert's Formula, mixed with licorice extract. Together, these herbs decrease gut inflammation, while stimulating non-inflammatory parts of the immune system such as Killer-T cells and interferon.

Cod liver oil (1 tbs. with each meal) is another old standby. With its Omega-3 fatty acid, vitamin A and vitamin D, the oil cools inflammation and helps to repair damaged tissue.

It is essential for CD patients to eat easily digested foods that are nutrient-rich. Telly ate steamed vegetables for the first five days, followed by systematically reintroducing foods into his diet, beginning with cooked fish and then pineapple core, rice and oats. The severe cramping pain disappeared after three days. After a month, Telly "felt like a new man": no cramping, no bloody or mucousy stools, and some weight gain. He soon learned that the pain would reappear if he ate raw or highly processed foods.

The digestion of a fruit or vegetable begins with its ripening in the sun and ends with stomach acid and pancreatic enzymes. Most CD patients are deficient in enzymes necessary for digestion. Accordingly, Telly took a supplement with meals consisting of a broad spectrum of enzymes. Of course, foods potentially contain the enzymes necessary for their digestion. These are the same chemicals that give a fruit or vegetable its color and taste. Since enzymes are created in the last few days of ripening, they are not found in produce picked green and allowed to "ripen" on the way to market, which is why a hothouse tomato has little taste compared to one that has been vine-ripened.

Enzymes are active within a narrow range of temperatures: from 102 to 110 degrees Fahrenheit. To promote digestion, the food should be heated at a moderate temperature, just until its fiber begins to soften. This is what happens within one's mouth, stomach and intestines when there is sufficient "digestive fire." Lacking the ability to thoroughly cook a food in one's body, one must digest it by applying heat from a stove or oven. You can see when a vegetable is fully heat activated because its color brightens.

Sometimes it is difficult for busy people to prepare good meals. This was the case with Telly, since his sales job demanded that he be on the road several days each month. In such cases, it is better to stir up a drink with a food supplement than brave a strange restaurant. Several experiments have investigated the benefits for Crohn's patients of consuming a supplement with pre-digested nutrients.[7] From such studies, we've learned that the best product for managing CD is the so-called "Elemental Diet" containing medium chain fatty acids. With it, gut permeability begins to noticeably improve within days. It is has been shown that CD patients without acute inflammation can safely withdraw from steroids when consuming such supplements.

Lacking the ability to thoroughly cook a food in one's body, one must digest it by applying heat from a stove or oven.

Once Telly's inflammatory markers receded, he was able to gradually withdraw from his medications. His physical health steadily improved, though we both observed his spirits to be down. Telly was feeling apprehensive that "at any moment everything might collapse." Such anxious depression is not uncommon for someone recovering from a chronic illness. Moreover, about one third of those with inflammatory bowel syndromes suffered depression before as well as after exhibiting bowel pathology.

Telly had recently experienced an incident in which a stranger had been "rude" to him in public. He suddenly felt so angry that he was unable to speak. This reminded me of three homeopathic rubrics: "overly sensitive to rudeness," "speechless from indignation" and "anger with indignation." *Staphisagria* is a plant-derived homeopathic remedy that is associated with these rubrics. It also has the unique ability to treat abdominal cramping and nausea caused by feelings of indignation so profound as to make one want to die. Immediately upon taking the homeopathic pellets, his face relaxed and I heard his colon gurgle.

Here was an opportunity: Telly's guard was down and his heart open to his own strengths and sensibilities.

"What does it take to become a world-class cyclist?"

"You fight and keep fighting. Sometimes you hurt, but you keep on peddling."

"Aren't there times when you push too far too fast?"

"Sometimes that's what it takes to get over the finish line first. Actually, there are guys competing who just go on guts alone. But they don't last long before their bodies break."

"So, it takes more than drive to be a world-class athlete."

"Yea, it takes a balance between a will to win and a sense of what your body can stand."

"Telly, I know that you're not competing now, but you can remember the feeling of balance that alerts you to when you're going too far in one direction or another?"

"Yea, the momentum keeps you on track and there's a gut feeling that tells you how far you can lean into a jump without falling."

"That also sounds like the feeling you've described about what makes for expert training."

"It's sort of like knowing the difference between a good soreness from stretching and the first twinge when you're about to go too far."

"Well Telly, I think that's the same sense of momentum and balance that will keep your health on track."

Three years later, Telly is engaging in friendly competitions and helping to train younger athletes. He periodically senses the beginnings of nephrosis or CD, almost always following a few days of heavy stress or holiday pastries. But the symptoms disappear in short order after returning to a healthy schedule. The ongoing process of maintaining balance provides a powerful reminder that he is in control of his body and mind. Meanwhile, with the birth of his son, Telly is busy charting a new history for he and his family.

CHAPTER FOUR

Relics and Fossils

Mementos of people and events can remind us of how to live well. They keep us close to the lights of home. But they can also make the move to a new and healthier life more difficult. When we hold onto remnants of the past that are no longer alive and life giving, we are left with relics and fossils. You may not realize for many years that something like the gnawed remains of an old fish are lashed to the side of your boat.

Ernest Hemingway was revered and despised for attempting to create a life independent from the people surrounding him. He took great pride in his Nobel-winning *The Old Man and the Sea* because it was his one story not derived from copious notes taken with a journalistic eye. Over the next ten years, Hemingway became increasingly depressed as he reflected on his inability to recapture that freedom of expression. The stories he constructed in those final years had derivative characters that stared back at him "as though from the morgue." In a discarded draft (which he saved) of his Nobel Prize speech, he wrote, "There is no lonelier man than the writer when he is writing, except the suicide. Nor is there any happier, nor more exhausted man when he has written well. If he has written well...he must do it again. There is always another morning and another morning."

Even Hemingway's early stories told with vigor have been desiccated by critics subscribing to the influence paradigm. They argue that his manliness in words and actions (e.g., his love for war, hunting, deep-sea fishing, prizefights and bullfights), was an over response to his love-hate feelings for his mother. Armchair psychoanalysis such as this ignores what is most centrally expressed in the Hemingway archives. (Like many other artists with a depressive bent, he was compulsive about preserving his observations.) In these reflections is explicated a conscious battle to assert his will over controlling forces: everything from Nazism to his mother's passive-aggressive behavior.

At the age of sixty-two and finding himself unable to write a few sentences describing the election of John Kennedy, Hemingway saw the forces of inertia gently and inexorably leading him to a state of decay and eventual randomness. He viewed his suicide, from a double-barreled shotgun to the head, as the last act of an enervated will.

There is great irony in that Ernest used the same shotgun to kill himself as did his father thirty-three years earlier. While Ernest obviously took his life into his own hands, he also conceded to what seemed inevitable. For many years, he had derived a sense of solace from that old shotgun hanging on the mantle. The family heirloom (a *relic* of sorts) was a macabre reminder of Clarence Hemingway, but also a potential avenue of escape.

Apparently, the Hemingway family took to heart this approach to solving problems, since Ernest's brother and sister also committed suicide. And in 1996, his granddaughter, Margaux, killed herself with an overdose of a sedative. That this followed from Clarence's legacy of action rather than genes alone is evidenced by there not having been inordinate numbers of suicides in previous generations of the family.

The comfort and meaningfulness of home is derived from the experience of sharing a collective narrative, even if the story is horrific. When others share your temporal landmarks they lend emotional support and increase the likelihood that you will continue to navigate those well-lit shores. Unfortunately, this perpetuates the illusion of safe movement when actually circling an area with Great White sharks and life-threatening rocks beneath the surface.

There are at least 30,000 suicides completed each year in America, and 200,000 unsuccessful attempts.[1] The mortality rate from suicide has consistently been higher than that from homicide. The rates are particularly high for young adults. For those in their twenties, suicide is contemplated most often by medical students, young physicians, and men with guns. In two-thirds of all suicide cases, it is seen by the perpetrator as the solution to depression.

The *reductionist* paradigm claims to explain a social phenomenon such as suicide at its lowest common denominator. As the argument goes, most "suicides" are depressed, and most of "the depressed" have low levels of the neurotransmitter serotonin; therefore, suicide is caused by low serotonin levels.

This syllogism is false. Because elevated or depressed levels of serotonin *accompany* a state of mind, does not mean that it *causes* that mental state. Even if depression could be experimentally induced by inhibiting serotonin, it would be a questionable extrapolation to the real world because there is evidence that serotonin levels can fall *after* depression of mood.

The above syllogism is also questionable because in many nervous system pathologies we know that an abnormal level of a hormone or neurotransmitter is necessary, though, by itself, not sufficient to cause signs or symptoms of the disease. This means that a number of factors must come together before illness results. Lastly, the syllogism is fallacious because the jingoistic "suicides" lumps within one normative category all individuals who have committed or attempted suicide, just as "the depressed" inappropriately equates all individuals who have been depressed. Members of the Hemingway family might have a gene that inhibits serotonin production or use, but this does not strictly determine depression or suicide without that individual adopting for his or her own the legacy of Clarence Hemingway.

Because of their simplicity, reductionist arguments are loved by most everyone. For example, I recently heard a group of "holistic" nurses applaud a lecturer who explained that it is easier for women than for men to live alone just as there is one ovum and millions of sperm. It is easier to substitute "just as" for causality, to ignore the choices made by individual men and women, to selectively attend to certain physiological functions while ignoring others (e.g., that for both men and women, testosterone is derived from progesterone, and estrogen is derived from testosterone), and to ignore the consequences of blindly accepting the argument (e.g., defining "manliness" by sperm count, or "femininity" by the number of eggs laid). Reductionist reasoning, while helping us to map out the details of a known area, prevents us from shifting paradigms and slowly desiccates the thought process.

Convincing rhetoric almost always begins with a conclusion that the audience wants to hear, typically supported by assertions that combine reductionist and normative assumptions. Where the reductionist paradigm establishes causality by building from the bottom-up, the normative paradigm explains a phenomenon by treating it as an example of a broader class. Whether it is the reductionist simile (e.g., "Packs of men are like so many sperm") or the normative metaphor of inclusion (e.g., "If you understand depression, you'll understand suicide), there is the assumption that the phenomenon in question has been influenced (either by its constituent parts or its environment). Unfortunately, with either extrapolation, our attention is directed away from the individual making critical decisions.

So, what do I recommend? Evidence. A movement that has the potential to shake up today's healthcare system is known as "evidence-based medicine." As a research psychologist turned medical student, I was shocked to learn that most of the medical doctors' standard of practice is passed on from teacher to student without the benefit of scientific evidence. By some calculations, only twenty percent of what is practiced is supported by rigorous clinical trials. In 2002 I reviewed the nearly 100,000 clinical studies indexed in Medline. There were less than 700 double blind, placebo-controlled clinical studies, out of which only 450 had demonstrated a positive effect from a therapy. More than half of the evidence-based therapies address the cardiovascular system. When looking at the research on cancer, we find that over the years there have been only twelve rigorously controlled clinical experiments demonstrating the efficacy of therapy and only one of these replicated.

Doctors become defensive facing the scarcity of evidence and counter that their armamentarium would be drastically reduced if they were limited only to therapies supported by controlled studies. I am not one to demean the traditional passing of knowledge from one generation of doctors to the next, except when what remains is a narrative stripped of meaning. Cortisone to manage chronic inflammation, Prozac for chronic fatigue syndrome, antacids for young children, childhood vaccinations for three-month-olds, the avoidance of eggs for hypercholesterolemia, the use of sunscreens to prevent cancer, these and countless other prescriptions are preserved only by the rhetoric of reductionist and normative assumptions. Someday, evidence from rigorously controlled experiments might prove that they have some worth or relegate them to the bin of lifeless relics.

Jerazad

I first met Jerazad at a gallery where she was showing her artwork. At the heart of the exhibit was a life size montage of herself, created out of handwritten letters. The silhouette highlighted her long hair and shapely body. After our brief introductions, she indicated that she had had cancer but was now in remission, and wanted an appointment to discuss her "health concerns."

What does it mean to a patient that her cancer has gone into remission? In my first consultation with Jerazad I learned that her oncologist had just told her that she no longer had signs of cancer of the breast and associated lymph nodes. She felt vindicated for refusing post-operative chemotherapy or radiation five years earlier, but was apprehensive that her body might be making more tumors. It takes between five and twenty years to produce a noticeable tumor, depending upon the type and location of the cancer and the state of the individual's health. Unfortunately, this leaves a great deal of uncertainty for the cancer victim to worry over.

Every one of us every day makes thousands of cancer cells, but a healthy body also manages its cancer production so as to prevent the development of a tumor.

To the physician "complete breast cancer remission" means that there has been no detectable recurrence of a tumor for five or more years. To the cancer pathologist, remission means that a patient now has less than one billion cancer cells. To either professional, remission does not mean that the person no longer has cancer cells, but only that the number is not sufficient to form a tumor. A patient weighing 150 pounds with a fast growing cancer, will produce more than 500,000 cancer cells each day, while someone who is "normal" or "cancer-free" or "in complete remission" produces about 120,000 cancer cells each day. Normally we are oblivious to our cancer cells until their mass becomes palpable or these eternally immature cells displace healthy ones that have a full life cycle, thereby depriving a physiological system of fully functional cells.

As with most cancer patients, Jerazad did not know why or how her body was making cancer cells, nor had she been counseled how to best prevent a recurrence. I explained that every one of us every day makes thousands of cancer cells, but a healthy body also manages its cancer production so as to prevent the development of a tumor. Most patients feel less victimized by their disease when hearing that cancer is something we all live with, much as we do the bacteria Streptococcus, E. coli and H. pylori, and fungi such as Candida.

Jerazad expressed interest in how the body fights cancer on a daily basis, and I explained that the naturopathic approach involves supporting each step of the process. The body's front line of defense is not killing cancer cells but rather converting them to healthy cells that grow up, perform their functions, reproduce and die. Such "differentiation" is the responsibility of the steroid hormone known as vitamin D3. If this conversion fails, the immune system is called on, at the bequest of vitamin D and melatonin, to kill cancer cells. And if eradication of cancer cells cannot keep up with their reproduction, a fibrous tumor is formed to wall-off the cancer cells from the surrounding healthy tissue.

Given that she had already had a cancerous tumor, it was likely that other cancer agglomerations existed at various stages of development. Since the surgically removed tumor had been estrogen-driven, the next one would most likely surface in a reproductive organ. In our discussion, we focused on the positive prognosis that she could prevent future tumors by strengthening her ability to manage cancer, and by making changes so as to eliminate the underlying cause of excessive cancer cell production.

Jerazad credited her quitting a stressful job as a college administrator and engaging in Tibetan Ayurvedic practices for protecting her in the years after the partial mastectomy. But much of her present symptomology suggested to me that she still suffered some hidden stress. She experienced severe PMS cramping pain, an irritable bowel alternating between diarrhea and constipation, and painful stomach ulcers. Her body constantly created fibrotic cysts in her breasts and the endometrium of her uterus. Her sleep was disturbed by nightmares of being raped and dying.

Jerazad had felt great fear when she first got the diagnosis of cancer. This quickly led to feelings of anxious depression that contributed to her divorce. Apparently her husband had been "controlling," though, like many cancer patients, Jerazad denied harboring any feelings of anger: "There is no place for anger in the practice of Tibetan Buddhism."

I further inquired into her early history. Jerazad had grown up in an orthodox Jewish family living in Iran. On the Jewish Sabbath, her family would draw the curtains so the neighbors could not see them perform their prayers. Of course their community knew that they were Jewish, but this was not a problem so long as they kept their practice a secret. When followers of fundamentalist Islam took control of Iran, Jerazad's family immigrated to America. She had certainly learned the schema for hiding unpleasantness within herself, and, failing that, the virtues of a timely escape.

I decided to not challenge Jerazad's tendency to secretiveness until we had established a trusting relationship. In general, it is best to not crack the cistern until you've created a channel for the water to flow.

For now, I felt it most productive to address her request for symptomatic relief of PMS and an irritable bowel, and to begin a program of naturopathic cancer prevention. Accordingly, I prescribed an herbal formula (with Black Cohosh) to alleviate cramping pain, cod liver oil to help with inflammatory symptoms and the regulation of cell growth, and a low glycemic, low acidifying diet. I also recommended that she should do aerobic exercise out-of-doors at least four days each week.

The first principle of naturopathic therapy and prevention is to stimulate and support the body-mind complex to heal itself. We know that vitamin D3 serves to differentiate cancer cells, and melatonin up-regulates the immune system. Jerazad could support vitamin D and melatonin production by walking or gardening in the sunlight (preferably without glasses) and relaxing in complete darkness twelve to thirteen hours later.

Certain botanicals increase the orderly reproduction of cells (by promoting cyclic AMP) and interfering with cancer cell reproduction (by promoting interferon). I recommended Panax ginseng because of studies showing that it induces cell differentiation by promoting both cAMP and interferon.

The body's primary antioxidant that helps prevent free radicals from becoming carcinogenic is glutathione. Vitamins C and E, the mineral selenium, and the amino acid L-Cysteine are the building blocks necessary for the production of glutathione. Some patients have a body genetically predisposed to use glutathione to protect itself from chemotherapy and radiation, in which case these nutrients should be prescribed with caution. Since Jerazad was not undergoing such therapies, I recommended that she supplement with C, E, and selenium.

The most important naturopathic principle for cancer therapy and prevention is to slow down cancer cell proliferation by eliminating its cause. This means (a) decreasing exposure to environmental toxins (e.g., smog, asbestos, PCBs), (b) avoiding adulterated food and water (e.g., oxidized corn or safflower oil, hormone-fed meat and dairy, charred meats, chlorinated water by-products), (c) decreasing consumption of cancer fuels (e.g., peanuts, high glycemic foods, the amino acids phenylalanine and methionine), and (d) developing non-suppressive coping skills.

I suggested that Jerazad join a breast cancer support group. There is good evidence that those cancer patients who take part in a support or therapy group have significantly fewer recurrences of the disease.[2] This is the case across different types of cancer and different schedules of therapy. These results make sense since cancer patients are generally more likely to deal with stress by repressing negative feelings. Women asked to write about their "deepest thoughts and feelings regarding [their] breast cancer" have a significant decrease in physical symptoms.[3] Writing so as to engage one's negative emotions significantly increases the number of WBCs, while thought suppression results in a significant decrease in WBCs.[4] Unfortunately, the patients who would profit the most from emotionally engaged journaling or a support group are the least likely to participate.

Jerazad left town soon after our second meeting, and I did not see her as a patient for the following three years. We would occasionally run into each other in Santa Barbara, when she would indicate that she was continuing her practice of Tibetan Buddhist meditation, and was feeling "fine." Breast cancer patients (relative to women without a history of cancerous tumors) are more likely to keep to themselves feelings of anger or grief. I suspected that this might be the case with Jerazad, given her schema of secretiveness. But in such cases, you can only quietly wait for the patient to emerge from the forest and share her secret.

When Jerazad did reemerge to consult with me, she was again "apprehensive" about her health. She had cancerous lesions in her right breast and accompanying lymph nodes, and a suspicious mass in the right lung. She felt some discomfort in the affected areas and was experiencing a lack of energy. It was apparent that a fundamental change would be necessary to turn her health around.

"Jerazad, you're amazing. If it were me, I'd be a lot more than apprehensive!"

She ignored the opportunity to touch her fear. "I had just returned from Brazil. I felt like a new person. The women there are so feminine; I felt free and we danced in the street. But all that didn't keep me from getting another tumor. My oncologist has recommended a complete bilateral mastectomy followed by chemotherapy."

"So, why do you think your body has continued to make so many cancer cells?"

"It's another estrogen cancer, so maybe it has to do with my being a woman. If I had more masculine energy then I might be OK."

"I'm trying to imagine what that would look like."

Laughing: "I guess having no breasts and no hair to start with!"

I asked her if she could feel the lump in her breast. She attempted to do so by poking her breast through her sweater with a stiff finger.

"Before the Brazil trip, when did you last feel really good about your body?"

"I was a pretty wild teenager after we got settled in California. That's when I found my soul-mate."

"Tell me about him."

"He was a young Israeli going to college here. He is my soul-mate, and so, after he returned to Israel, we shared our deepest feelings in letters for the next seven years. Eventually, I saved money enough to fly there and surprise him. At his home, he introduced me to his wife and children before excusing himself. I spent the next hour looking at the family album."

"You must have been livid that the man you thought was your soul-mate would deceive you like that."

"I pretended that we were just friends and bought a return ticket to Los Angeles. I took all those love letters and made a poster of myself."

"I remember seeing it. So, you kept it all those years and through all your moves?"

"It's my best piece of work. Everyone loves it."

"You know what I think everyone loves about that montage: the real woman it represents. Do you still have the thing?"

"Of course. Maybe I should give it to one of my friends."

"You know Jerazad, sometimes we can create rituals that are the most powerful of medicines. Your attachment to that piece of art has made it a relic, and it's keeping the woman it portrays from letting go of the past and fully growing up."

I had spoken my mind, and Jerazad was neither ready to torch the montage nor undergo surgery, so we proceeded with developing gentler aspects of a health plan. We worked out a diet that would fit her needs as well as a few nutritional and herbal supplements (including Panax and Maitake mushroom extract). We also considered some physical therapies that she could apply to her breast and lymph nodes. An old naturopathic technique for alleviating pain and inflammation while bolstering the immune system is the application of a castor oil pack. The patient wets a cotton towel in castor oil, applies it to the disturbed soft tissue, covers it with a wool cloth and a heating pad or hot water bottle. After a few minutes, even severe pain can be dramatically reduced.

An important principle of cancer therapy is to deliver therapeutic agents as close to the target cells as possible. For the past twenty years, DMSO has been found to serve as a carrier of chemotherapeutic agents, including retinoids such as vitamin A.[5] Vitamin A, and DMSO itself, are substances known to make cancer cells mature into benign cells. As a polar solvent, DMSO is absorbed through the skin, along with the vitamin A, until it penetrates cancer cells and begins the process of differentiation. Jerazad was eager to give it a try, and so I informed her of two possible problems: (a) because of its sulphur content, DMSO makes patients smell like garlic, (b) DMSO will transport *anything* in contact with the skin, so that cleanliness is essential. She already ate a lot of garlic and she would be careful to gently wash the areas of application.

Soon after beginning the physical treatments, Jerazad reported feeling much better. She considered this to be "tough love for her breast and lymph nodes." It appeared to me that she began to groom herself with an eye to looking more feminine.

But perhaps most significant of a change of heart occurred one midnight when Jerazad asked an old friend to help her "dispose of some history." With a little moral support, she was able to burn the montage. When I saw her two weeks later, she was experiencing a greater sense of energy and was much more expressive of her feelings. In fact, she was on her way to Switzerland to be with a man she had loved for the past three years. I was feeling an apprehensive *deja vu* when she added "This time *he's* paying for the tickets!"

Marsha

I was a very cautious medical student, and therefore grateful to spend most of my internship under the supervision of Dr. Drew Collins, a naturopath noted for diving into uncharted waters. One evening he asked me to examine a middle-aged woman who had come to the clinic suffering from "irregular menses." The most salient feature about Marsha was that while offering a thorough health history she at no time mentioned the scar on her left arm.

The scar was leathery, at least a centimeter thick, and extended several inches across the lateral side of her elbow so as to prevent her from straightening her arm. When I asked her how it had come about, she replied that she had been in a car accident as a young girl, but that she could not recall any of the details. It didn't bother her, and she had refused plastic surgery to correct it. Dr. Collins asked me to perform acupuncture around the perimeter of the scar. I did so and scheduled Marsha for a follow-up visit the following week.

She returned quite upset. All around the edges of the scar it had started to pink-up, indicating that blood was returning to the area. It was sore, and the return of some mobility to the arm was disconcerting to her. Even more troublesome for Marsha was the sudden occurrence of dreams of the old accident. It was as if bringing her mummified arm back to life had released images hidden therein, what many people call "muscle memory" or "body memory." The events leading up to the accident were now clear. Her teenage brother had taken her for a drive and had stroked her breast. She had screamed and clutched her chest, and a second later a truck crushed the driver's side of the car. In her dream she sees herself impacting the windshield. While her brother had died, Marsha had suffered cuts to her arm and face.

I ran into Marsha about six months later as she waited to see another physician. She took me aside and, with the gravest sincerity, informed me, "There are things that shouldn't be touched until you're ready. My arm can move, but the rest of me is stuck seeing and hearing those horrors." I apologized for not respecting her enough to wait until she was ready, and asked if she had thought about psychotherapy. For Marsha, the problem with therapy was that it would demand her thinking about the accident, when what she wanted was to forget. Since I soon left to start a practice in Santa Barbara, I don't know if Marsha ever got to the place where she could work through her terror.

When I recall this case, it reminds me that having the tools to open someone up is not the same as knowing what to do with the secret that lies within. It is the therapist's job as guide to look for submerged rocks, hidden debris or subtle currents that the patient cannot or will not see. Sometimes we see rapids ahead; other times the patient is in a period of relative calm when we barely notice any movement at all. Our role may be to simply remind that it is time to fasten the life jacket, or, if stuck in stagnant waters, to help unfurl the sails.

Are there pathologies better left alone? Certainly there are instances when it is better to get off the boat and register at the Holiday Inn! I heartily recommend Carl Jung's autobiography *Memories, Dreams, Reflections*[6] to all those studying the healing arts. Herein we see illustrated the importance of knowing one's own limits before attempting to expose someone else's psyche. In one example, Jung was mentoring a medical doctor with the intention of the latter becoming a psychoanalyst. Jung explained that in order to serve others the physician must begin the psychoanalytic process himself. Despite protestations that his was "the most normal of lives," they began discussing the physician's dreams. After some weeks, he had a dream loaded with emotional content. In it, he was wandering about a strange medieval building, when he stumbled upon a gigantic, darkened chamber. After some exploration, he discovered, sitting in the middle of the room, an idiot child of about two years old who had smeared itself with feces. Jung realized that "here was a latent psychosis! I must say that I sweated as I tried to lead him out of that dream." He then proffered the most innocuous interpretation of the dream possible, and began discussing an earlier dream that could be interpreted as meaning that he should no longer pursue psychoanalysis. Jung reflects that both he and the budding therapist were relieved when the latter gave up psychoanalytic training.

Lila

Both "relic" and "never well since" schemas sharply demarcate one's life narrative. When relic memories are cherished or comprise an integral part of our identities they create a vortex from which it is particularly difficult to escape. Oh, how we cling to the memory of an old love! Perhaps the memory relic lies in a song felt with perfect promise, or in a crumble of petite Madeleine dipped in lime tea, or the willow blue mug that was your father's. Or it may be the pair of old shoes you know lie under the bed that still carry the scent of your late husband. Such mementos seem to flesh-out our memories so that we are once again sensing the lost moment in time.

In reality, no one can revivify a past event in all its diverse aspects. Rather, we selectively attend to only certain characteristics of the past, often with the assistance of sensory mementos. We do not hold onto the past so much as anchor ourselves in its vicinity with memory relics devoid of real life complexity. Lila's case illustrates how certain images call for us to relive them, while others are so traumatic that we hold them too close to see.

Lila was suffering with feelings of stress, daily headaches, and irritable bowels. She had nightmares of her own death. She was sharply dressed, quite thin, with a silicon "platform" and facial implants, and skin that appeared overly tanned seen next to the platinum colored hair. Lila was proud that in her twenties and thirties she had been a "trophy wife." This evoked for me images of a sculpted piece of tin that requires constant polishing, or the remains of a beautiful fish strapped to an aging fisherman's boat. I was wondering who would willfully turn themselves into a relic.

After Lila was divorced, she met a man "who loved her for herself." With feelings leaving no room for doubt, they were soon married and checked into a Las Vegas Hotel. He went into the bathroom to take a shower, slipped and died instantly from the resulting concussion.

The tragic loss left Lila with an image of herself as cold and hollow as a mirror. With her loving relationship shattered, Lila was left with her trophy schema, and acquiesced with a vengeance. Burying the memory of her lost love, she experienced the intensification of symptoms that had existed prior to the accident. While always short-tempered, Lila could no longer stand the presence of her daughter and granddaughter, and was taking Xanax each night to reduce anxiety. What had been periodic headaches were now daily migraines, which she was barely managing with codeine and high doses of Tylenol. Where she had experienced a "sensitive bowel," now she suffered painful bouts of gas and constipation. Where she had always been "lean," since the accident she had become anorexic, losing weight and bone mass.

Lila had recently developed a number of symptoms suggestive of impaired liver detoxification. Alcohol, caffeine, codeine, Fosamax (prescribed to prevent bone loss), and aromatics such as gasoline and perfume triggered severe reactions, including aggravation of her headaches and bowels. Such chemicals put a load on the liver and cause pathologic symptoms when the detoxification process takes too long to neutralize the poisons. She experienced a peculiar metallic taste in her mouth, also consistent with holding toxins.

I recommended that she gradually decrease exposure to the above chemicals and start a diet that would promote liver detoxification and restore bone mass. To the "liver detoxification pathway diet" described in Chapter 3 (see Frances) we added, for bone support, non-fat yogurt and European black currants. For nutritional supplements, I recommended two daily doses each: 500 mg natural vitamin C, 400 IU natural vitamin E, 400 mcg folic acid, and a mineral formula with hydroxyappetite and magnesium to help replace bone. Given her anxiety level and difficulty sleeping, I recommended that just before bed, Lila take half a teaspoon of glycine mixed in a glass of elderberry juice or oat milk. Glycine is an amino acid essential to the conjugation detoxification pathway, and serves as a neurotransmitter that promotes muscle relaxation and sleep.

I also recommended three traditional herbs for the purpose of moistening, easing bowels, assimilating nutrients, and promoting sleep: lotus seeds, and a tea of Eclipta and cooked Rehmannia. The seeds are very tasty, and the tea is pleasantly sweet.

It was essential that Lila start exercising on a regular basis. Walking each morning to the point of mouth breathing would help expel toxins. Weight training is a requirement for restoring bone mass; even high potency, high quality, mineral supplements will do nothing unless you give your body the message that they are needed. The bone loss that Lila has experienced is the consequence of both low nutrient intake and anxious depression for which her body is cannibalizing its resources. Fortunately, aerobic and resistance exercise both relieve depression, improve appetite, and build self-confidence.

After a minute of reflecting on the protocol, Lila anticipated numerous problems with its implementation. The diet would require that she cook for herself, the herbs would require explaining to the local herbalist what she needed, and exercise would mean changing her lunch break to an earlier hour. I pointed out that each of these actions would involve her taking positive steps for her own welfare. Changing course in life with respect to promoting personal health requires asserting to one's community that henceforth you value yourself enough to implement self-serving behaviors. For Lila, this would mean setting new priorities, discussing the implementation of new behaviors with her daughter, granddaughter, and boss (a spa administrator), and accepting the consequences of those actions.

Changing course in life with respect to promoting personal health requires asserting to one's community that henceforth you value yourself enough to implement self-serving behaviors.

Changing one's pattern of behavior creates a vortex of attention from all involved. Typically, one's decision is initially challenged: the person who resolves to stop smoking will be offered cigarettes, or your ex-husband will call once you've decided to "move on with your life." It's helpful for health-care professionals to alert patients engaged in such heroic efforts that once they have resisted the temptation to inertia and are clear about their resolve, the social vortex that remains will support their decision. Johann Wolfgang von Goethe wrote, "[T]here is one elementary truth…that the moment one definitely commits oneself, then Providence moves too. All sorts of things occur to help one that would never otherwise have occurred. A whole stream of events issues from the decision."

Lila, like most folks with whom I discuss this topic, objected to "parading my selfish behavior in front of everyone like dirty laundry."

I pointed out that "Doing things that are good for yourself is generally a good thing for those around you, especially people who love you. After all, how can you care for someone else if you are too weak to help yourself? Once you respect your own needs, a boss or family member is more likely to accommodate your wishes."

I think this was the first moment that Lila really looked at me, and I felt no need to fill the silence. The look of *Are you crazy?* began to melt into the memory *I can love and be loved*, when she suddenly excused herself "to the little girl's room to powder my nose."

A shift in worldview is a tall order for anyone. Except for the blissful weeks with her late fiancé, Lila had viewed the actions of people as being controlled by those in a position of power. When not able to overtly exert her will, she could always seduce by making herself into something desired.

However, the death of a loved one, or facing one's own mortality through a serious illness, provides a window of opportunity for fundamental change. Over the following two months Lila gradually implemented her protocol. The change in behavior was reinforced by the diminishing of headaches and irritable bowel symptoms, and by the increasing respect she was afforded. For example, her boss allowed her to arrange work hours so as to take a long, vigorous walk in the late morning. As she gained some weight, I complimented her on looking good, strong, flexible.

We discussed the ongoing power struggle between Lila and her daughter who would neither be bullied nor seduced into submission. This was becoming less of a problem as Lila established rules regarding her personal space in the house and the hours she needed for herself. Four or five days each week, she was cooking healthy meals for herself to which her family was welcome to share (or not). Four days a week she did weight training, progressing in a two-month period from four-pound to eight-pound dumbbells. Lila's daughter had shown some interest in what it was that so engaged her mother.

Reconnecting with her daughter had its dangers, since it meant being drawn into her ex-husband's circle of trophy friends. Until she had been replaced by the new wife, Lila had served the function of entertaining this collection of "beautiful" men and women. In fact, those very skills made her an invaluable employee at the spa. One evening some months later, I saw her in town with one of "the circle." Lila had four-inch heels, a short skirt, a blouse leaving little to the imagination, and make-up stiff enough to inhibit the expression of emotions.

I found it encouraging that Lila made another appointment with me and that she was disturbed once again by headaches and irritable bowel symptoms. This time, she was clearly more motivated to make fundamental changes. We laughingly referred to her search for identity as "getting off the mantle" or "recycling the trophy," but eventually settled on "shedding skin."

With modest encouragement, she used her "drive to survive" and chameleon skills to obtain a different job and arrange for her daughter to move out. "Living alone won't be easy, but I think I like the feeling of being independent." She returned to the diet and exercises of the old protocol, and her symptoms quickly decreased in frequency and intensity.

It had been seven years since her newlywed husband died, and, now alone with her feelings, Lila experienced grief.

"You know what? I've thought about that man every minute since his passing, but this is the first time I've cried."

"Did you picture or feel the two of you together, like it was then?"

"No, I thought about Jim, but I could never bear to think of us doing things together."

"Sometimes your tears can bring memories to life."

With a tear running down her face, "Yeah, but it hurts to have those memories."

"It will stop hurting so much pretty soon, but you'll probably be surprised every once in awhile by a twinge of memory."

"I still have his old clothes in storage. I've been afraid to open them. Some haven't even been washed."

"You know what Lila? Cleaning out the closet does not mean forsaking someone. By the way, what do you think you might discover in that memory of yours?"

"There may not be much *to* remember since we hadn't known each other very long before getting married. I guess I'm afraid I'll feel empty."

I reassured Lila that she was in an excellent space to begin psychotherapy, and that it would be very exciting to see with what she would fill "the trophy." We agreed that the challenge would be for her to remain aware of the direction her choices led, be it acquiescing to widowhood or "trophydom," nurturing an independent self or creating a loving relationship.

Celeste

Sometimes love transmutes, for example into respectful familiarity, so slowly that the changes aren't noticed. Or we may choose to redirect our loving energy to someone or something new. But when the object of our affections is suddenly withdrawn from us, we may hold the painful memory as though embracing a Saguaro cactus in full bloom. By focusing on the fateful event, we relegate the preceding period of "bliss" and the subsequent period of loneliness to the periphery of consciousness. With time, the feeling of abandonment typically fades, leaving a hollowed-out cactus and an occasional needle-like twinge. But in order to engage a new relationship, it is sometimes necessary to either clear out the dead wood or start planting seeds in more fertile soil.

Celeste came to me to work on a number of complaints: a total cholesterol level of 255, a low level of thyroid hormone, occasional headaches felt behind the eyes, "extreme emotional stress," and a swollen middle finger. She had always been athletically inclined and practiced the Tai Qi sword once or twice each week. Now, in her late fifties, she appeared emaciated with dry skin and dandruff; she had cold extremities; under her tongue, the blood vessels appeared purple; her blood and heat pulses were barely palpable. Also consistent with a *Vata* imbalance was an ongoing problem of gas, bloating, and stomachache.

I explained that her elevated LDL cholesterol was probably a function of the body's attempt to produce sufficient thyroid and stress hormones. Having a low thyroid aggravates dry skin since the hormone is instrumental in replacing skin cells, and it can cause indigestion because it manages metabolic rate such that a decrease slows digestion. Meanwhile, to the extent that one lives in the sympathetic nervous system "fight or flight" mode, one directs energy away from the process of digestion and the regeneration of tissue. For example, calcium, magnesium, and vitamin D are used for *both* the laying down of bone and the creation of stress hormones such as serotonin and adrenaline. Celeste eventually revealed that she had become self-conscious of her mouth since, despite consuming plenty of minerals, she was breaking teeth at an alarming rate.

The vicious cycle here is that feelings of stress deplete the body of nutrients necessary to cope, which, in turn, aggravates digestion, thereby inhibiting the assimilation and use of those same nutrients. At the same time, losing teeth makes digestion more difficult and generally increases stress levels. Most likely, Celeste's level of serotonin was being severely taxed, given that the neurotransmitter/hormone has the two jobs of relaxing the mind and promoting digestion by bringing blood to the intestines.

Celeste had been contentedly married for thirty years, until her husband, Roger, announced that he was in love with another woman and that he would be moving out immediately. Celeste could live in the house and take care of his mother. During the four months since then, she could not concentrate her mind on much other than replaying the moment when her life had been changed.

I asked Celeste about what contact she still had with Roger, and she indicated that he was around most days, visiting his mother, changing clothes, and getting this or that tool from the garage. I asked if she expected to get her husband back. She answered "No, he seems quite happy just the way things are." She thought it a good idea to set some boundaries about when he would come to the house, and to ask him to transfer his personal effects to his new home. Several months later, with divorce proceedings underway, I was pleased to hear that Celeste had announced a yard sale, provoking Roger to finally remove his stuff.

While driving in Celeste's neighborhood, I noticed a particularly ugly Saguaro standing sentry in front of her otherwise lushly gardened house. At our next consultation, she indicated that Roger had planted it there many years ago. Just knowing that it was there made her angry, but she was "not ready to let it go." Soon, we were both chuckling at her swollen middle finger, the proportions of which resembled Roger's cactus. When it would flare up, Celeste referred to her finger as "Roger." Ironically, she had no anger or second thoughts about continuing the care of Roger's mother. Celeste appreciated the company and was not about to displace her well-maintained anger onto a woman in need.

We met once a month over the following year. I recommended that she eat regular meals and add more deep-sea fish to her diet. She began to take a walk out-of-doors on her noon hour, and to practice Tai Qi on a daily basis. To support the production of thyroid hormones, I recommended an organic thyroid supplement.

For her cholesterol, Celeste took an Ayurvedic resin with the strange sounding name of *guggulu* (*Commiphora mukul*). *Guggulu* is a yellow resin from a tree closely related to myrrh. It was prescribed by the ancient Indian physician Charaka as a rejuvenative of the nerves and a help in moving energy (e.g., morning arthritic pain from lack of movement). Modern science finds that it cleanses the blood of excess fat and LDL cholesterol by boosting blood levels of HDL and increasing the free flow of blood and lymph.

Ayurvedic practice puts a premium on *pranayama* (Sanskrit for breath or energy control). Modern science confirms that (a) different mental and physical states are associated with different breathing patterns (e.g., acidosis is associated with short, rapid breaths), and (b) altering one's breathing will change one's mental or physical state (e.g., long, forceful exhalation through the nose rapidly alkalinizes).

As a complement to the *guggulu*, I taught Celeste a *pranayama* exercise traditionally used to calm the mind, burn fat, move lymph, and raise energy. I demonstrated the following steps, to be performed in the morning and evening, sitting upright or standing: (1) slowly inhale through the left nostril (closing the right nostril by pressing with a finger), (2) hold the breath for a moment before slowly exhaling through the right nostril, (3) hold a moment before inhaling through the right nostril, (4) hold a moment before exhaling through the left. Ideally, the inhalation, holding, and exhalation

will be of the same duration; this can be facilitated by silently count-
ing to one's self, or reciting a mantra or statement of affirmation.
(More elaborate breathing patterns are sometimes recommended,
but I find that it can become too distracting.) Four such breaths are
usually sufficient to calm the mind.

An integral part of Ayurvedic medicine is the use of food to
maintain balance or correct a pathologic state.[7] In Ayurveda, an
ideal diet to maintain health is one that includes all six tastes: sweet,
salty, sour, pungent (hot), bitter, and astringent. Biochemically, each
of these tastes comes from a food with a different profile of essential
nutrients, the totality of which provides a balanced diet. According
to Ayurvedic theory, in order to help modulate a disorder in which
Vata has come to dominate, one typically includes more salty and
less bitter foods. This was perplexing to Celeste, since in following
public health warnings she had been for many years emphasizing
bitter greens while avoiding salt! I explained that each one of us has
a unique set of needs to optimize our bodies and minds. Once she
had rebalanced herself, then she could eat as much bitter with as little salt as she liked. Celeste felt relieved that she could now salt her
vegetables without feeling guilty.

From an Ayurvedic perspective, Celeste was deficient in *Pitta*
(digestive "fire") and *Kapha* (moisture and tissue mass), and so I recommended that she also include foods tasting of sour or sweet. She
even craved certain foods that combine both tastes, for example,
lemonade, yogurt with honey, and sweet and sour fish. For the most
part, there is agreement between evaluations made by Ayurvedic and
modern Western medicines. For example, Celeste had abnormally
high pH levels (one cause of her poor digestion) that could be lowered with the addition of acidic foods, which typically taste sour or
have the effect of raising blood sugar.

After the first four months of therapy, Celeste's thyroid hormones had normalized, her LDL cholesterol had lowered ten percent, her HDL had risen twenty percent, and her digestion felt "very
much improved." Periodically, her finger inflamed and she felt
stressed. The Saguaro was still standing.

Now that Celeste had experience making meaningful life

changes and in the process developed a trusting relationship with me, we resumed our discussion of her life prior to the fateful abandonment by her husband. I asked her to relate to me her earliest memory or dream. Despite taking my request seriously and "sleeping on it" for a week, Celeste could not recall any specific experience before she was six years of age. She intuited that before then "everything must have been good."

In her personal narrative, there had been an early landmark event separating a time of blissful ignorance from a subsequent period of loneliness. Her father had "walked out on the family," and in subsequent years her mother had paid for her to be kept by a woman in a nearby town. Celeste's mother would occasionally take her out, but would introduce her as "my little friend." I asked Celeste how she had felt. After a little thought, she answered, "I remember that the other women had *their* children, and that I felt envious." For me, the most salient feature of this poignant story was how Celeste told it. She had tears (one in particular running down her left cheek) without breaking expression or pausing in her delivery.

At this point I was struck that the totality of Celeste's symptoms are consistent with the homeopathic portrait known as *Lycopodium*. The *Lycopodium* personality sees his or her life demarcated by an inadvertent expulsion from paradise. They are envious to the point of tears of those who have what they seem to have lost. Physically, they appear old prematurely, and get ill (with forehead pain and digestive disturbances) when forced to take steps to change their lives before they are ready. The *Lycopodium* mind becomes sharpened from taking a meandering walk in the open air.

Unlike the double-blind, placebo controlled experiments on *Lycopodium* in which subjects are unaware of the homeopathic remedy selected, I tendered the above portrait as a possibility. Unlike other homeopathic portraits that I had suggested over the months, Celeste strongly identified with *Lycopodium*, and was amazed that so many of her characteristics belonged to the portrait. I gave her a single, high potency, dose of *Lycopodium* while she sat in my office, and suggested that she find time each week to "take a walkabout."

The next day, I received an e-mail from Celeste, saying that she felt "clearer and stronger" than she had in years. Her feeling of well being was very much evident when I saw her a month later; she had even decided to visit her mother. The idea was for Celeste and her daughter to take a meandering drive across six western states, arriving with a few days to spend with "mom."

The following month, I learned that the trip had been uneventful: no special adventures or resolution of family history. However, Celeste's daughter appreciated their peaceful time together, "Our relationship moved to an easier, more adult level even though we had little to say to my grandmother."

I continued to meet with Celeste over the following months, doling out occasional doses of *Lycopodium*. She steadily gained weight, and her skin appeared less dry. She recalled early dream-like images of her parents that were "less than idyllic." On some reflection, Celeste recalled that her mother would "shush" her to keep her father from getting annoyed. Viewed through the lens of adult sensibilities, it seems that her mother had directed her marital frustrations at Celeste, who then unwittingly took on guilt for the broken marriage. In relating this to me, I saw, for the first time in Celeste, her expression of grief complement her tears.

In our last meeting, Celeste related that she was having romantic feelings for someone. She was also eyeing the chainsaw in the garage and the Saguaro which was now close to falling over of its own dead weight.

There are at least five different approaches to explaining how homeopathic *Lycopodium* might have benefited Celeste. 1) Her improved sense of wellbeing was merely coincidental with taking the homeopathic remedy. 2) A simple placebo theory is that she must have been highly suggestible to feeling better and that the "remedy" provided an avenue to that suggestion. 3) A psychological theory (e.g., that of Gestalt psychology) might hypothesize that reflecting on her various physical and mental characteristics as an integral whole provided a simplified and hence more meaningful personal identity, thus yielding the phenomenal impression of improved well being. 4) Homeopaths are likely to view her reaction as an example of "like-cures-like" since full doses of *Lycopodium* elicit in healthy subjects all of Celeste's pathologic symptoms, while highly dilute doses have been found to mobilize the body-mind complex to heal itself. 5) Naturopathic physicians take a more pragmatic point of view: homeopathic *Lycopodium* will be accepted as useful whatever its mechanism of operation to the extent that the existing evidence has been well researched.

I find constitutional homeopathy to be an interaction between doctor and individual with the goal of self-discovery. Homeopathic portraits provide a broadened perspective, much like an aerial view of the various facets of one's self partially obscured by patches of fog. What seems, when lost within its muck, an endless swampy bog may actually be essential to the life and flow of an unseen estuary. Having an incomplete map makes life an ongoing exploration. That we are constructing a map as we go allows that an estuary or a vast tidal plane may lie just out of sight, becoming revealed or further obscured by the decisions we make. A homeopathic remedy gives one a sample taste of what a whole self-portrait would look like. When well selected, it tantalizes just enough to motivate you to move ahead.

CHAPTER FIVE

Ghosts, Gods,
and Haunting Refrains

A personal belief might be the echo of a significant person's voice without our being aware of it. Recognition of such mental tapes, as they are happening, is critical to successfully freeing one's self from the past. But how does one begin to replace the haunted vaults of one's mind?

The words *ghost* (from Old English *gst*) and *spirit* (from Latin *spiritus*) are both derived from words for breath, being an invisible force escaping from the center of one's body. In ancient times and across many cultures, the meaningful control of the breath (i.e., the voice) was a magical means of communicating with the spirit of anything that could be named. It is interesting that the English word *voice* comes from the Latin *vox*, originally meaning to summon.

The Jivaros of the upper Amazon basin still engage in battle with neighboring tribes and exercise their skills at shrinking the victim's head into a trophy called a *tsantsa*. Their skills at war and biotechnology are conducted at the bequest of family ghosts. In fact, every event in their environment is believed to have been caused by a ghost or some nature spirit. In their system, people can be instrumental in causing ill by ignoring the ancestral voices, or by failing to summon the appropriate ghost or spirit. Psychologist Julian Jaynes has argued that the ability to reflect and intentionally organize one's own actions is a relatively recent evolutionary development.[1] Supposedly, at the time when *The Iliad* was poetry and song, people would receive edicts from the "gods" directing their actions. But, by the time of Homer's *Odyssey*, man was willfully defying the gods, of course at his own peril. With the gradual transition from unconscious to willful actions, fewer and fewer people spoke directly with the gods, and with their passing came a nostalgic longing for "divine volition" that could only be partially satisfied with codified laws of behavior. Such divine edicts may have sounded similar to the voices that Frances (Chapter 3) obeyed, ignored with the help of medication, and missed after she had detoxified.

The desire for divine volition certainly has not left modern Homo sapiens. Whether it is the trance state of a Jivaro shaman or a sophisticated Catholic prayer, the hope is to relinquish one's will. Witness the fervent prayer of St. Ignatius: "Take, Lord, and receive all my liberty, my memory, my understanding, and my entire will, all that I have and possess. Thou hast given all to me. To Thee, O Lord, I return it."

Martin Luther argued that the will is impotent to promote good, and did so with such vehemence as to leave his stigmata upon philosophical discussion for nearly 500 years. In *The Bondage of the Will*, he writes "it is apparent that 'free-will', even in the noblest men, not only does not possess and cannot effect anything, but does not even know what is righteous in God's sight…God reveals the righteousness of salvation…to men who sit ignorantly in darkness."[2]

In *The World as Will and Idea*, Arthur Schopenhauer argues that wherever we have thought of God as above, behind, or within the matter or experience of the world, we should think of human will. Despite his substitution of will for God, Schopenhauer viewed the will as bondage and an instrument of pain as much as had Luther or Buddha. He wrote, "The only purpose in life must be escaping the will and its painful strivings."[3]

It is unfortunate that twentieth century philosophers, taking their lead from Schopenhauer, have also failed to free their discussion of the will from arguments surrounding God's will. Sometimes will is viewed as an action based on observation and reason (as did Luther), in other instances, will is desire and physiologic need (as viewed by Schopenhauer), but the discussion inevitably devolves to whether we can act freely in a world programmed by God, genes, or environmental influences.

In every age, there have been men and women who have turned their lives around by renouncing the assumption that the world's programming must be their own. The success of this heroic venture depends upon the ability to discriminate the inner voices programmed by others from the ongoing development of one's own voice.

Mileva Einstein-Maric is an enigma embedded within nineteenth-century sensibilities, wrapped within the contemporary women's movement. She was born in 1875 in what is today Serbia, studied math and physics at the Federal Polytechnic in Zurich, and became Albert Einstein's first wife. Though obviously talented and playing some role in the discovery of Special and General Relativity, Einstein-Maric dropped out of academia, an ephemeral figure hidden in Albert's shadow past. Over the past thirty-five years (though especially since 1992), Mileva has been the subject of four biographies, two plays, two novels and countless speculation as to the exact role she played and why she so dramatically turned away from her personal career.

To some, Mileva is the modern day Lilith (the first wife in Paradise, cast out by Adam): a brilliant mathematician who was a full partner in the development of Special Relativity, whose contributions were all but forgotten as Albert's passions roamed elsewhere. It is even reported that the original manuscript submitted for publication, and eventually responsible for a Nobel Prize, was authored jointly by Einstein and Einstein-Marity (a Hungarianized version of Maric).

As a child, Mileva showed talent for mathematics and music. Her father, an upwardly mobile civil servant, aspired to have his children receive an education suited to developing their potentials. As such, he repeatedly pulled political strings so that Mileva could study math and science. She became one of the first girls to attend Hungary's Royal Gymnasium, and one of only five women enrolled at the Polytechnic. In their school years, Mileva and Albert each spoke romantically about their joint study of relative motion. A few years later, Mileva defended her husband's action to delete her name from the publications, asserting "We are 'ein Stein,' one stone!"

Albert's letters show that his infatuation faded after their marriage, and thirteen years into it, he described Mileva as "a typical woman who wants nothing more than to suck a man dry." At this point no one dared to suggest that Albert's theories had been a collaboration. In 1919, Albert divorced Mileva so that he could remarry, and she was awarded the interest from his Nobel Prize. For the remainder of Mileva's life, she tended her sons and grew progressively more melancholy, dying of a stroke in 1948.

In contrast to the Scorned Woman theory, some of Einstein's biographers obviously subscribe to the Great Man theory. Mileva is viewed as a possessive woman, jealous of her husband's genius and notoriety. After their first year of courting, Mileva left to study at the University of Heidelberg. The story is that she could not resist Albert's brilliance for more than a semester, returned to Zurich in order to catch him, and thereafter was content to possess what *Time* magazine declared "The Person of the Century." Once she had latched onto Albert she had no further personal ambitions, and what scholarly abilities she had had simply vaporized.

A third, Social Suppression, theory argues that Mileva was a victim of her culture, in which women were expected to subjugate their careers and creativity to the interests of their family. She grew up in a small nineteenth-century eastern European village, wherein acculturation was reinforced by countless slogans. The cultural voice echoing in Mileva's mind told her "A good woman loves her husband and children more than her own life." Her mother often reminded her, "Better to know how to behave than to have gold."

None of these theories does justice to Mileva (or any individual for that matter) because each attempts to account for the events in her life by a limited selection of forces, and because each theory is searching for critical *influences* that drove her away from an intellectually productive life. Certainly, Mileva had a *variety* of inner voices telling her what to do, including an emerging sense of her own will.

Some of those voices told her it was good to live through Albert's accomplishments, and to support her husband against all criticism. For example, by 1910, Mileva was overworked and fatigued trying to maintain her family. When her physician suggested that Albert needed to work to support them, she rose up and pronounced: "Isn't it clear to anyone that my husband works himself half dead? His thirst for knowledge, his search for ever newer understanding, his work, this is his genius."

Other voices, for example those reflecting her parents' wishes, told her to value her intellectual accomplishments over the promise of romance. Contrary to traditional Serbian culture, both her father and mother took great pride that men respected their daughter's scientific opinions.

Mileva could slip into the voice of her mother, especially when chastising Albert (who was almost four years her junior). From Overbye's *Einstein in Love*:

Albert: "There was this old whore…"

Mileva: "*Albert!*" [Said with a stomp of the foot.][4]

There were also times when she spoke or wrote in a way that echoes the voice of Albert in his more Bohemian moments. For example, when a friend had just had his heart broken, Mileva wrote Albert: "But it serves him right, why does he need to fall in love nowadays?"

Of the correspondence capturing the various voices of the young couple, the ones that sound most true to their hearts and their youth are those between "Johnnie" and "Dollie," playful pseudonyms used by Albert and Mileva.

My dear Johnnie,

Because I like you so much, and because you're so far away
that I can't give you a little kiss, I'm writing this letter to ask if
you like me as much as I like you? Answer me immediately.

A thousand kisses from your Dollie[5]

The pseudonyms freed them from the necessity to sound pro-
fessorial, self-sufficient and in control of their emotions. Dollie,
more than Mileva, spells out her feelings with childlike simplicity
while showing her emotional vulnerability and neediness.

There is a *never well since* event in Mileva's life that is ignored by
the theorists. When Mileva left Zurich for Heidelberg, she was at
the head of her class in math and physics; on returning a semester
later, she was then and thereafter at the bottom of her class. In spec-
ulating as to those decisions that changed Mileva's life, we are faced
with the daunting task of reconstructing a mind that functioned a
century ago. While, of course, it is impossible to interact with
Mileva, time yields a broadening perspective on her motivations.

The University of Heidelberg was more prestigious than the
Polytechnic, though it did not give women students credit toward
graduation. It may have been attractive to Mileva that she did not
know anyone in Heidelberg. At the age of twenty-three, without the
distractions that Albert (at the age of nineteen) and his friends were
offering, and removed from the judgments of family and friends, she
could perhaps find her *own* voice.

In a letter to Mileva while she was in Heidelberg, Albert proffered, in a cool authoritarian voice that only a twenty-year-old can
muster, that she might write him if she got bored. From the distance
of Heidelberg, Mileva responded with a voice that is at once ambiva-
lent, flirtatious, witty, and ironic.

"...you said I shouldn't write until I was bored — and I am
very obedient...I waited and waited for boredom to set
in...and I'm not sure what to do about it. On the other
hand, I could wait until the end of time, but then you would
think me a barbarian — on the other, I still can't write you

with a clear conscience." [Heidelberg, 1897][6]

In the Spring of 1898 Mileva returned to Zurich, for the most part because of her infatuation with Albert. Unlike Mileva, Albert always sounds self-assured. In a typical letter, Albert apologizes for neglecting Mileva and immediately begins to relate his latest brilliant idea. Neither Albert nor Mileva ever appear to doubt that his ideas would be important to science.

Believing that one's emotions go unheard is a commonly cited cause for depression, and Albert had little patience for problematic expressions of the heart. Mileva had a great deal to consider but no one with whom she could share her distress. Little was said between the couple about their first, illegitimate child, Liesserl, while the practical decisions of what to do with her fell upon Mileva. There was also the problem of Albert's mother who did not hide her disdain for Mileva. Albert's advice was for the couple to avoid his mother as much as possible, including any public expressions of affection that might be communicated to her. Later, when married, Mileva seemed to have brooded over the choices she made that led to abandoning her personal career.

What made their marriage bearable for thirteen years was that both Mileva and Albert shared an interest predating their pursuit of physics, namely their love for music. Albert had played the violin since before he spoke complete sentences; he carried it around with him in his knapsack. Mileva, by the age of seven, could read music and play the tamburica, a lute-like instrument from Asia; throughout her adult life she also played the piano. The two loved to play music together, or one would sing while the other played. Even in times of their greatest animosity, they would speak of each other's beautiful voice, and tenderly touch that empty space in their heart.

Crystel

We all accommodate the people with whom we live, sometimes without thinking, sometimes as a reasoned compromise, sometimes as a means of survival. Even years after their passing, we continue to hear their voice as our own, speak so as to express their wishes, and perform actions reflecting their continued presence. This might mean continuing to sleep on the left side of the bed, or sitting at one side of the dining table even after your spouse has long departed. Or continuing to pad about quietly, not thinking that that behavior no longer serves to maintain your late husband's peace of mind.

It is common to perpetuate hand-me-down beliefs that do not represent one's own voice. Such hauntings often sound like the voice of authority: a controlling parent or spouse. "Don't turn on the fountain; it uses too much electricity." "Don't flush the toilet; it will fill the cesspool." "Your head is wet; you'll catch your death of cold." I recently caught myself, alone in my study, saying "sorry" to a lamp after bumping into it, though I have no recollection of having been instructed as a child to apologize even to people.

Ghosts often manifest as idiosyncratic overgeneralizations. For example, this afternoon at the local airport I was privy to both "*No one* checks in their luggage," and "*Everyone* checks in their luggage." Exaggerations offered with the voice of authority indicate that either the speaker is under too much stress to express himself rationally, or the beliefs were acquired under circumstances when critical thinking had not developed or had been suspended.

The death of a loved one is the event that results in the greatest amount of stress in our lives. As discussed in an earlier chapter, twenty-eight percent of breast cancer cases are diagnosed within a year of an event that causes grief. The risk of illness is compounded when the loss is of the very person who has provided intimate emotional support. A depressed nervous system means a depressed immune system since the same chemical messengers that serve the nervous system also maintain immune function. Short-term, the biochemical effect of grief is to allow the person to continue life-sustaining functions without being overwhelmed by sympathetic nervous system discharge. In fact, a moderate amount of stress is anti-inflammatory and serves to delay onset of pathological symptoms. Long-term, the depressed production of neurotransmitters makes the person's immune system less responsive, and, consequently, his or her physical well being vulnerable to attack.

Crystel is a pretty though wan-looking woman in her late for-ties, with a manner of expressing herself that belies both a cultured upbringing and a hypervigilant mind. She breezed across my con-sulting office, sitting in the chair the furthest to my right. Crystel had suffered with stress, fragile teeth, and bladder infections for the previous two years. She was presently in the midst of a bladder infec-tion and was also experiencing pain in her right side that appeared on examination to be a flare-up of shingles.

Interstitial cystitis typically involves an overgrowth of bacteria that results in inflammatory reactions such as swelling of tissues that make the passage of urine difficult and painful, while increasing the urgency to urinate. A vicious cycle ensues, in which the inflamma-tion discourages one from drinking fluids, which, in turn, allows bacteria to grow undisturbed.

As is the case with stomach ulcers (see Chapter One, *Inertia, Change and Choice*), there is a vicious loop that stretches between emotional stress and a chronic bladder infection. Antibiotics will fail to permanently reverse cystitis so long as there is unresolved stress, since there is always some amount of bacteria that can soon propa-gate to pathological levels. Crystel had completed several series of antibiotics, though with only temporary relief. In fact, it was becoming progressively more difficult to eradicate the latest bout. This is understandable in that each antibiotic series leaves behind a colony of bacteria more resistant to antibiotics than its deceased comrades. Moreover, the history of failed attempts to cure Crystel's infection was itself creating apprehension and additional stress.

An experiment published in *The Journal of Urology* induced stress in subjects with and without interstitial cystitis and looked at the resulting manifestation of symptoms. Twenty-five minutes of working on a timed mental test significantly increased pain and uri-nary urgency symptoms in the cystitis patients but not the control subjects. For the cystitis patients, both pain and urgency increased in intensity from the beginning of the stress test to seventy minutes after its completion, after which symptoms gradually decreased to pre-test levels.[7]

Crystel had numerous physical signs of stress. Weight loss, bone loss, shingles, and chronic cystitis all follow from living under stress for far too long. I asked her, "So, what happened in your life before you got all these diseases?"

"Oh, I was happy and studied and played the piano and hung out with my family at holidays; all the normal things of life."

"Yes, but did something happen about two years ago when you started getting sick?"

"I guess...I mean yes...You really want me to talk about it?"

"Please."

Her jaw tightened. "Death. I've been sitting in dark churches burying the only people I love. My mother cared for me whenever I was sick like no one else. My father has already got another woman, and I'm suppose to call her 'Mom'."

"Who else had died?"

Looking down toward her feet: "My boyfriend went shortly after my mother. Some kind of rapidly growing tumor."

"Crystel, I know you are upset. I can see it in your body. Could you describe what you're feeling right now?"

Pointing to her solar plexus with both hands: "A dark tunnel."

"Take a deep breath...hold it...and just let it out."

"I feel fear...like moving down a dark tunnel."

We sat for a minute before I asked her to tell me more about her boyfriend.

Laurence had been her "one and only love," the only man with whom she had ever had sexual relations. He was more than twenty years older than Crystel, and they had lived together for about ten years.

"It sounds as though their illnesses and deaths came without much warning?"

"Who knows when someone is going to leave us."

In response to this rhetorical question, I thought it best to bring her back to the present. "So Crystel, how do you spend your time now?"

Her jaw closed tight before responding. "I'm now going to do whatever it takes to feel better...I know he's going to leave everything to *that* woman. Once I get my health back, I'll take care of it."

Of course, it wasn't just *anyone* who Crystel had lost, but the very sources of her inner loving voice. And her mother and boyfriend had not just left her, but had suddenly died. And her father could cut her off from financial resources that she had always relied upon. She was stuck, wavering between blissful memories of the past, suppression of the thought that her loved ones are gone, anger that her financial resources are now out of her control, and staring helplessly at the entrance of an abyss.

A strictly allopathic approach to Crystel's emotional pain would distract her from the darkness and encourage her to experience new sources of joy. Here, we would find classical (Pavlovian) and operant (Skinnerian) conditioning therapies, or recommendations to get a cat or listen to popular upbeat songs. On the other hand, a homeopathically-oriented therapist would use that dark tunnel as an entrance, and support her in her journey through it. Here, we would find cognitive-behavioral and psychoanalytic therapies, or perhaps journaling while listening to the Blues.

It sounded to me that Crystel was subject to different mental voices: one sounded lofty or ethereal, another was a vulnerable child, and a third was a no-nonsense take-charge voice. When there is one or more "ghosts" speaking through the patient, we may use the voice as our guide into the tunnel. I mustered my most authoritative, take-charge voice, tightened my jaw and declared in words reflecting her own, "I know you have a problem with stress causing interstitial cystitis, herpes zoster, and osteopenia. We can take care of it."

Crystel closed her eyes, and when she opened them again, there were tears. She smiled prettily and asked, "Should I worry that you will leave me with all my problems?"

This is an example of *psychological transference*, wherein the patient acts toward the therapist as though he is a significant person from his or her past. Crystel is directing her fear of abandonment toward me just at that moment when I have assumed her voice of authority. Apparently, Crystel fears that the speaker of that voice will eventually disappear, just as happened to Laurence or whomever else imprinted the voice upon her. She clearly does not realize that the voice is one of her own ghosts.

I answered her while attempting to stay with the authoritative voice: "Crystel, I promise you that I will meet with you for the next few Tuesdays. There are some things you need to do during that time, including changing what you eat, reducing stressful thinking, and doing some soul-searching."

For most meals, Crystel was eating a diet of comfort foods that featured almonds, chocolate, graham crackers and potatoes. We discussed how the herpes virus underlying shingles is fostered not only by stress but certain foods. Chocolate is the most common food trigger, almonds feed the virus the amino acid L-arginine, and high glycemic foods (e.g., chocolate, crackers, potatoes) depress the immune system. She would have to get her comfort from other sources. I recommended coconut milk soup that she could get at a Thai restaurant or make in her own kitchen. Coconut milk is sweet and rich without raising blood sugar, and high in short-chained fatty acids that support the immune system. Crystel also agreed to drink more fluids, especially licorice tea. Licorice is sweet tasting, helps build interferon (to interfere with viral replication), and gives a boost to the adrenals.

Cystitis can progress to a kidney infection if left untreated, and Crystel made it clear that she would not take pharmaceutical antibiotics. Accordingly, I recommended that she add to her cooling tea, four times each day, a drop of the essential oil of sandalwood and a drop of thyme oil.

Essential oils are necessary for plants to fight bacteria and fungi, and can act as antibiotics for humans as well. An essential oil is easily recognized in a living plant because it is also responsible for its scent. Only the purest forms and smallest amounts should be consumed, since more than the recommended amounts will cause die-off reactions such as headaches and diarrhea. Using both sandalwood and thyme oils, most types of bacteria and fungi known to overgrow the urinary tract will be destroyed. Sandalwood is used in Ayurvedic medicine for any urinary inflammation, but more generally as a way of calming the nerves and "hot" emotions such as anger.

For the next five days, Crystel would apply alternating hot and cold compresses to the area between her naval and urethra: a hot towel for four-to-five minutes immediately followed by a cold compress for one minute, immediately repeated twice more. This brings blood circulation to the area and relaxes the urinary tract, thereby facilitating healing. In general, ailments with a strong psychosomatic component respond particularly well to physical therapies that stimulate the parasympathetic nervous system. Physical healing takes place to the extent that one rests in a parasympathetic mode. Moreover, such therapies move one's awareness from the realm of obsessive thoughts to sensations of the body. Making one's self aware of dynamic, relaxing sensations in an area of the body that had been locked away in fear, validates a patient's ability to escape the tyranny of the mind.

In general, ailments with a strong psychosomatic component respond particularly well to physical therapies that stimulate the parasympathetic nervous system.

I instructed Crystel in a *pranayama* technique in which she would breathe in slowly through her nose, hold her breath for a few seconds, breathe out slowly, hold, etc. On the out-breath she would make a soothing humming sound. She could feel a relaxing sensation on trying it in my office, and felt that it would work even better when she was alone.

The following Tuesday, Crystel arrived twenty minutes late and seemed relieved that I was still there. As we entered my inner office, she once again walked briskly the length of the room; I could envision her being escorted by an invisible hand to the farthest seat.

Her shingles pain and burning bladder had both receded considerably, and she had gained confidence in her protocol. While taking her pulses, I asked her to recount her earliest memory, even a dream, and she replied that she couldn't recall anything specific before she was seven years of age. As she explained this, I noticed that her breathing became short and shallow.

"I guess I'm sort of afraid to remember what happened that early. I do recall having something like asthma that would come on when I'd get nervous."

I moved around behind Crystel and asked her to begin her breathing practice. After a couple of slow, deep breaths, I suggested that she simultaneously raise her eyes on the in-breath and lower them when breathing out. She almost immediately went into a light trance.

"Crystel, your mind has the ability to show you anything. You may wonder what your mind will present to you when you're ready to see it. So, just breathe normally: relax it in and out. And let your eyes and voice relax into the darkness. You will let me know that you understand something by simply raising one of your fingers."

Her right index finger rose.

"When you are quite ready, you will see a young girl with dark hair, but only when your mind is ready to do so." After a minute, I saw Crystel's finger lift. Her breathing became more of a pant and I could hear a faint wheeze. A more allopathically-oriented hypnotist would, at this point, ask Crystel to reframe her imaginal experience so as to picture herself breathing easy. I decided to use the *vulnerable child* voice to enter the "tunnel" and help her explore.

"I don't know where we are; do you?"

A raised finger.

"I'll stay close." Crystel's breathing normalized, and I decided to be quiet.

After a few minutes I opened the imaginal door for her to wake up: "When you have explored this space as much as you need for now, you will begin to be more aware of the sounds about you, the sunlight coming into the office, the feeling of your own breath falling lightly on your lip. You feel rested and will remember what you've seen."

In less than a minute, Crystel took a deep breath and looked at me. For the first time, her pulses were regular and strong.

I asked her, "So, where did we come from?"

"I recall my mother angry with me, saying 'You have quite a mouth!' And my father being comforting and very gentle and loving. Then, I remember him putting something in my mouth. And it was hard to breathe."

"Do you know what the 'something' was?"

"You know, it's what every woman hates to do."

Crystel obviously recalled an incident of sexual abuse. The generalization about women suggests an attempt of the adult Crystel to express the confusing feelings of a child. I thought a moment about how to challenge Crystel's overgeneralization without being dismissed as "a man."

"By the way, I think that's not true for all women. But you were a little girl. A few moments ago, when you were picturing all this, how did you feel about it and about your father?"

Crystel took a deep breath and moved her chair so as to sit directly in front of my desk. Her voice was neither that of a young girl nor a deeper voice of authority, but that of a reflective adult: "I felt love, and I liked it."

"And how do you feel right now?"

"I don't know. Maybe guilty, maybe angry. I don't know exactly. Strange, I feel calm about all this, as though I had known about my father and me all along."

"Do you think anyone else, your mother for example, ever found out what was going on?"

"I think so. Yes, by the time I was seven something happened and Dad stopped coming into my room. He didn't give me any special affection after that."

"What kind of feelings did that leave you?"

"I was angry with him and jealous of my mother. Pretty sick, heh?"

"Not at all. Your mother and father put their little girl into quite a bind. But I'm looking at the woman, and I see a person who is doing remarkably well with some difficult feelings."

Over the ensuing months, Crystel gradually became less

dependent on our relationship. At the same time, she was able to further explore and develop her own voice. Meanwhile, her bouts of cystitis almost disappeared, her bone mass increased, and she was enjoying the first stages of a relationship with a man her own age.

Maria

Nowhere do ghostly voices become more evident than when they hail from competing lovers wooing a childlike self that knows it *only wants to be loved*. Under such circumstances, one's own voice, other than its expression of desire, might be heard as a whisper, but can readily become smothered by the lovers' proclamations. Relinquishing one's own will, and the responsibility it carries, becomes most compelling when listening to voices singing the promise of love.

Maria came to my office asking for help with recurrent bouts of psoriasis, and advice to assure a healthy course of pregnancy. In her late twenties, Maria walked purposefully, presented dark, clear skin, and did not yet show evidence of the second trimester through her skirt and jacket. As Maria described her health history, I was impressed by her use of English idiom expressed with a handsome Italian accent.

During pregnancy, there is an increased physiological need for all nutrients, but especially for those that help to regulate growth. For this reason, I recommend a special vitamin formula, which, taken twice a day, provides sufficient amounts of vitamins B1 (2 mg), B6 (3 mg), and Folic Acid (8 mg). Like most things, more is not better: megadoses of vitamin B6, often recommended for morning sickness, can cause neurological damage to the fetus.

Pregnancy puts the mother at risk of acquiring diabetes, especially when there is family history of the disease (as is the case with Maria). The mother produces high levels of glucose for the benefit of the fetus. At the same time, because maternal insulin is not transported across the placenta, she experiences symptoms of low blood sugar (e.g., hunger and light-headedness). It is not advisable for her to replace glycemic foods with protein-rich foods containing more fat, because such dieting may induce high levels of *ketones*, which impair fetal brain development. In order to stabilize blood sugar levels, I recommended that Maria eat as many small meals as she pleased, of what she pleased.

Sixteen weeks into her pregnancy, Maria was still experiencing nausea and occasional vomiting, as do seventy percent of pregnant women. Though it is commonly called "morning sickness," pregnant women report nausea occurring throughout the day. It is a good example of how unpleasant symptoms can serve the body. Maria was pleased to hear that nausea and vomiting is associated with *decreased* risk of miscarriage, preterm birth, or low fetal birth weight.[8]

The most common aversions during pregnancy are to the taste of alcohol, or the smell of coffee or fatty meats, each of which can increase the liver's detoxification load. It has been hypothesized that this reaction causes the pregnant woman to physically expel and subsequently avoid foods that could cause birth defects or induce an abortion.[9] In fact, pregnant women who vomit suffer significantly fewer miscarriages than those who experience only nausea.

We next discussed a skin condition that Maria had lived with off and on for the past two years. Psoriasis shows up as a red rash with sharply demarcated borders, and is suffered by three percent of Americans. Lesions develop in areas where skin cells begin to divide as much as one thousand times the normal rate, producing silvery scales of cells.

The physiology, biochemistry, and treatment of psoriasis is a good example of how Ayurvedic medicine views the etiology of disease in general. When one's digestive "fire" is strong, nutrients are broken down in an orderly manner, yielding a feeling and appearance of vitality. But, when digestion is poor, undigested food becomes toxic, manifesting in irregular bowels and, eventually, lesions on the outer surface of the body. Psoriasis patients typically suffer from incomplete digestion of protein in the stomach, which results in toxic by-products being reabsorbed by the intestines, and a toxic load placed first on the liver and then the skin. Eventually, skin cells take to excessive reproduction in proportion to the demands placed on the system to eliminate waste.

I explained to Maria that managing her psoriasis in the next couple of months would improve her chances of having a trouble-free pregnancy. In the third trimester, the pregnant woman's cortisol levels rise, and with it an increased risk of generalized pustular psoriasis. This form of psoriasis spreads across the body and can even kill the mother and fetus.

I recommended that Maria get her necessary sixty grams of protein primarily in the form of liquid, pre-digested protein. This would help with the psoriasis without aggravating her nausea. If Maria had not been pregnant, I would have suggested that she take cod liver oil, as vitamins D and A, and omega-3 fatty acids serve to reduce inflammation and regulate skin cell growth. Fortunately, we know from many studies that patients with psoriasis respond well to moderate amounts of ultraviolet light, which causes the body to produce its own vitamin D. Because Maria's lesions were on her buttocks, she would sunbathe for thirty minutes each morning in the privacy of her backyard.

Since poor digestion is a causal factor in psoriasis, and digestion depends upon a relaxed parasympathetic state, it should not be surprising that anxiety or depression can precipitate psoriasis lesions. One medical review found that thirty-nine percent of psoriasis cases had a precipitating "never well since" event just prior to the initial episode.

I asked Maria whether anything special was going on in her life before her first bout with psoriasis two years ago. She paused for a moment and then shared her dilemma.

"The problem is that George, my husband, is such a fine man. There couldn't be a better husband. He makes no demands. My family in Florence loves him."

"Maria, this does not sound like a problem."

She turned to look in my eyes, "Dr. Reynolds, it *is* a problem. I met a man that has real passion: he looks at me like he's going to eat me up! For more than a year we just talked, but such talk! I was so torn between George and Tony that I created a room for myself."

"Do they know about each other?"

"George seemed to get more and more depressed trying to figure it out, until I finally told him."

"And the baby is…?"

"I don't know for sure; it could be George's or it could be Tony's, but I guess I hope that it's Tony's."

"It seems to me that you have a full plate: a job at the University clinic, a developing child, a passionate lover, and the best husband one could be estranged from! The skin lesions are a superficial reminder that there are problems on the inside. And not many people would even notice. My concern for your health, and that of your baby's, is that you listen to your heart."

"I don't really know what I feel. When I'm not working, I'm talking with my family on the phone, or hearing George make appeals, or Tony making plans. I know that I should make a decision, but I just can't."

"Due to your changing hormones, over the next year you're going to become more focused on your baby and even less inclined to make demanding decisions."

In the third trimester there is a dramatic rise in progesterone levels. Progesterone stimulates serotonin and GABA receptors that serve to relax the expectant mother at the cost of impaired cognitive functioning. In one survey of pregnant professional women, over eighty percent reported unusual forgetfulness, and over half reported difficulties reading. Such maternal amnesia persists for several months postpartum, during which time progesterone-to-estrogen ratios return to normal.[10]

I suggested to Maria that she could use the changes in her body to help discover what was most at her heart. After a couple of months, her changing hormone levels would make the competing voices less interesting.

"When that happens, Maria, you will be able to hear your own voice."

Maria let out a deep breath. "It's already too much to think about."

"Is there anyway that you can get away from both George and

Tony for the next couple months? That might give you a breather and some perspective."

"That's what I tried to do by taking my own bedroom; but it doesn't stop the barrage of questions and promises. And there would be other problems."

"Such as…?"

George is already depressed; he'd probably get really jealous. And Tony would want to move in. And, if I were alone, I wouldn't know what to do with myself."

"For right now, let's imagine that you don't have people competing for your attention. Take a deep breath, hold it for a moment, and just relax it out. With each breath, let yourself relax even deeper. Feel how your breath falls onto your upper lip, and allow your mind to wonder what it might see or feel when it is relaxed."

Maria's stomach gurgled and we both smiled.

"Maria, how do you feel alone with yourself?"

"Right now I feel good. I've almost never been alone. I come from a big family, and in my job I listen to other people's problems."

"Take a moment and consider what would happen if you explained to George, Tony, and maybe your family, that you need time to yourself, time each day when you wouldn't be available."

"George would take it as confirmation that I don't love him; he might get more depressed. Tony says he must be with me or at least talk to me every day; he probably wouldn't agree. My family would just call at a different time."

"Maria, when have you felt most like yourself?"

"George and I used to speak to each other in Italian about everything in life. Now, even when making love, it's in English. I can almost hear him translating into English!"

"Are there other times you feel like yourself?"

"When I climax with Tony I feel completely myself. He doesn't even seem to be there."

So far, I'd heard three distinct "ghosts" expressed by Maria. There is the voice that speaks in generalities, for example, an unconditional declaration of her husband's worth. From Maria's comments, it appears that this voice echoes that of her parents'.

There is also the plaintive cry of not knowing what to do. This voice seems to echo her husband's inability to hold onto his emotional center. Finally, there is the voice, obviously associated with Tony, which advances direct declarations of desire. It is likely that each of these people, in reality, have a more complex repertoire of voices, and that Maria is selectively focusing on certain personae to speak for her.

To my ear, Maria was speaking without her surrogate voices after she had done the little relaxation exercise and was contemplating how it feels to be herself. She agreed to set aside two hours each evening, when she would practice breath awareness, followed by journaling her thoughts and feelings.

Two weeks later, Maria brought in her journal, a large-format, hardbound book of unlined pages. She had initially recorded (in English) the times of her daily sunbathing, what she ate in each of her five meals, and interactions with George, her family, and her "boyfriend." Maria was pleasantly surprised that George felt all right with her taking time to herself. She speculated that this arrangement decreased his apprehension about telephone calls that would otherwise come from Tony. For his part, Tony responded by making more proclamations and demands. As anticipated, her family in Florence easily arranged to call in the morning instead of the evening.

"So, that leaves *you*, Maria. How did you feel having time to yourself?"

"At first I was bored. Then I listened to some music — old folk songs I heard my mother and father sing. And this week, I've enjoyed just sitting. In fact, I can feel my baby for the first time."

Over the following months, Maria maintained her morning and evening hours for herself, and filled her journal with pastel drawings of the significant persons in her life. George became more self-reliant and a good candidate for fatherhood. When Tony stopped returning Maria's phone calls, she was initially upset, but soon appreciated the freedom. Her psoriasis disappeared and has not returned. Most of all, Maria enjoys how her little girl smiles back at her.

Frank

Ghostly images are not only imprinted on us by figures from our youth, but are shaped from our own hand and animated with every breath we give to them. Of course, one may actually create something he dearly loves, only to have all but its memory disappear. Such a loss may continue to haunt one's life regardless of what is subsequently created. In Frank's case we find that the intention to make one's self whole has a seemingly magical power to ground one in the very reality that is sorely missing. We are granted a look behind the wizard's curtain, and discover real magic!

Frank came to me as a forty-six-year-old scientist with few physical or mental symptoms, but wanting a homeopathic approach to self-discovery. His pale skin, white shirt, and laboratory jacket merged together, leaving just a pleasant smile. I asked how he felt and he illustrated by going limp in the chair. Frank had multiple responsibilities and long hours. When I first met him, he was a full-time civil engineer, a full-time medical intern, a full-time husband, and a full-time father to eight children! A lecturer's voice would put him to sleep within seconds. On the verge of completing medical school, Frank was looking for a way to integrate the various parts of his life.

I explained that in constitutional homeopathy we search for what lies at one's heart, nurturing the growth of one layer of the personality after another. The initial layer is often related to boundaries. One's physical, psychological or social-psychological boundaries may cause problems, particularly when they are (a) unbending (rigid or fibrous), (b) excessively accommodating (fragile or porous), or even (c) illusive.

In the physical domain, pathological boundaries might manifest, for example, as atherosclerosis, sinus congestion, psoriasis, or a leaky gut. Psychological pathology manifests rigid boundaries as repression of emotions and instincts, while weak boundaries are found in those who act out their unconscious motives all too easily. In practice, overly rigid psychological boundaries may be indistinguishable from weak boundaries; for example, either may be responsible for blindly following a conditioned response. Moreover, both rigid and weak egos are more vulnerable to trauma than those that are flexible. In the social-psychological domain, we may view as pathological those who (a) indiscriminately acquire the emotions and beliefs of those around them (accommodating), (b) intentionally misrepresent themselves in order to exploit other's vulnerabilities (illusive), or (c) automatically hide their feelings and beliefs from public scrutiny (illusive).

It was apparent from our initial discussion that Frank held contrasting "voices": a physical weariness that cries out for nothing but rest, and an inner voice appealing for creative expression. He also had an inner world that was well hid from the public. Outwardly, Frank appeared soft, slow to act, and mild mannered to the point of being self-effacing; inwardly, he was brilliant and hard driving. In practice, there is no way of determining the strength of someone's boundaries other than observing how they respond to challenges encountered in the course of life or intentionally presented by the therapist.

A number of homeopathic drugs embody contrasts within the same person, especially remedies derived from minerals or from substances with a high mineral content. The portrait of homeopathic oyster shell calcium (*Calcarea carbonica*) epitomizes physical weakness and slowness in conjunction with a hidden wealth of ideas. The *Calcarea* personality will work to maintain a low profile within his social institutions while he unobtrusively organizes his thoughts into creative gems. Frank, for example, gave up engineering at the very time he was being recognized for his contributions to that profession. I mentioned to him that Charles Darwin and Albert Einstein each were content to hide within a public institution while they leisurely developed their theories.

The *soft* part of the *Calcarea* person does not want to be disturbed from his or her inertia, and without the structure of a regular job or family life, might never come out into public. For this reason, they are more comfortable with children than adults who might "blow their cover." Of course, *Calcareas* can be awakened if light is suddenly turned on them or their comfortable raft unexpectedly runs into rapids. After leaving his job as a patent clerk and becoming a very public figure, a disgruntled Albert Einstein wrote that he would have been forever content with the job of a lighthouse keeper. Charles Darwin leisurely worked on *The Origin of Species* for over fifteen years with no end in sight until he discovered that Alfred Wallace's manuscript on evolution was soon to be published. So provoked, Darwin concentrated his energies and produced in the following six months his theoretical "pearl."

Frank placed a few pellets of *Calcarea* under his tongue, looking much like an oyster consuming a grain of sand. He was pleasantly apprehensive about what might eventually be produced.

When I saw Frank the following week, his general sense of tiredness had turned into a feeling of "various weights dragging me down." He very much wanted time without the "burden" of dealing with patient problems or issues surrounding friends of the family. He said that he was "saving up" his energy in order to carry out his various responsibilities. His blood pressure was alternating between abnormally low and elevated; his cheek had broken out in brownish patches. These symptoms are indicative of adrenal hormones drained to the point where they barely keep one going. It struck both of us that the homeopathic *Calcarea* had opened his "shell," exposing a very tired man.

Frank had uncovered a portfolio from twenty years ago. He thought I might be interested in his first love, sketching. Frank obviously had had some talent. The ink portraits were technically adept and captured in just a few lines a real depth of expression.

In the homeopathic process, once boundary issues have been addressed, new symptoms may emerge from the exposed inner layer. Frank's feeling of being dragged down, his desire to be unburdened from the emotional baggage of strangers, his need to marshal his reserves of energy, the signs of adrenal insufficiency, and his early love of ink drawings, are a combination of characteristics unique to homeopathic *Sepia* (India ink).

The cuttlefish is a deep-sea mollusk that is phosphorescent when alone, though it spews out a cloud of ink to hide from other creatures, even from members of its own species. The ink consists of calcium salts and melanin. Melanin is responsible for skin pigment and is chemically related to adrenal catecholamines.

The tube in my hand held a few drops of highly dilute, homeopathic *Sepia* as I suggested to Frank that perhaps he too hid his "inner light" from prying eyes; this would be understandable, since such behavior would help him to avoid further responsibilities. He mustered a dignified smile and sighed, "You don't know the half of it," and then opened his mouth to new possibilities.

A few days later, Frank came in wearing a dark, conservative suit with dress shirt and tie. He was openly disgruntled about various people and things not performing as they should. In one week he would officially take on the role of physician. "But, my family and staff are not up to it," he said. "Which means that I am forced to see that everything happens on schedule. All I expect is for people to do their jobs." He was also disturbed that his digestion was not "what it should be" given that he always eats a good diet. In describing these responsibilities and "shoulds," Frank had tears in his eyes.

The new symptoms that Frank exhibited are strongly suggestive of the homeopathic remedy known as *Lycopodium*: tearfulness, critical about people not doing their job, distress from changing careers, distress from following a schedule, dressing so as to look highly competent, and the assumption that he should be healthy because he lives a virtuous life. Homeopathic *Lycopodium* is derived from club moss spores, a primitive organism growing in northern latitudes that has remained unchanged for the past 350 million years. For hundreds of years it has been the basis of fireworks, and used by shamans and stage magicians to create a puff of smoke for dramatic effect.

The *Lycopodium* personality is methodical and feels at his or her best when allowed to establish their own pace. They think most clearly when taking a leisurely, meandering walk in the open air. I smiled as Frank suggested that we continue our consultation walking outside.

Lycopodium personalities believe that if they had been left to their own devices their life would have been complete, even stately. Somewhere in their past they had been forced off, or at least distracted, from "the path." I asked Frank if this were the case, and he immediately shared that he had had a first wife and child. Contrary to his personal beliefs, they divorced and he completely lost contact with them. Ever since, he had been quietly haunted by this loss.

We continued to meander about, discussing how, where possible, it is better to implement new behaviors than to take a pill (even a homeopathic pill). Frank decided to give himself unstructured time and take a walkabout every day.

Two months later, Frank freed up a week or so to take a meandering drive across America, ostensibly to find *Lycopodium* moss. He drove from Arizona to Utah and Colorado, then east to the Atlantic, and south to northern Florida without finding the plant. (To really find club moss one would have to go to Canada.) Not wanting to return home empty handed, he got off the freeway, determined to at least purchase a bottle of homeopathic *Lycopodium* pellets. At the local health food store was a lazy-Susan display of homeopathic tubes. Frank struck up a casual conversation with the person on the other side of the display. The young woman had recently broken up with her husband and, like Frank, was driving across America "looking for something" when she too had decided that a homeopathic remedy might be the solution. In a few moments, Frank realized that the woman was, in fact, his first daughter!

Frank related this magical reconnection in a casual manner while introducing me to the latest member of his family. He added with a circumspect smile, "I never did get the *Lycopodium*." Frank, never mind the pellets; you got the magic!

CHAPTER SIX

Perfection

Anything worth doing is worth doing right. An anachronistic voice such as this is acquired early in life, and can either drive one toward excellence or to the point where he or she is afraid to make a move. Perfectionistic thinking makes some students excel and others too indecisive to choose a course of action or unwilling to submit their work unless it is perfect.

The word *perfect* comes from Latin *perfectus* meaning completed, and *perficere* meaning to perform completely. It is used as a noun ("perfection," "perfectionist," "perfectionism"), a verb ("to perfect") implying the best possible action, or an adjective describing the ultimate thing or event of its kind. Of the eighty movies with "perfect" in their title, most are adjectives tinged with irony. For example, *The*

Perfect Storm can kill you, and *The Perfect Husband* is bound to disappoint.

There has always been the implication that the road to perfection goes through pain. In medieval alchemy, "to perfect" a substance meant purifying (sublimating) it by fire. It would be dissolved, heated until evaporated, and then distilled. In the process of achieving spiritual "gold" one must first enter "the dark night of the soul" and then apply the "fire" of will and imagination so as to sublimate animalistic desires and fears into ecstatic pure love.

Psychologists describe certain characteristics common to perfectionistic thinking: (a) the belief that there is a right way to do things, (b) the application of a precise set of criteria for success, that causes one to (c) focus down onto a level where one is most likely to control the outcome, and (d) rarely, if ever, feeling satisfied about one's performance. This schema is often responsible for unproductive behavior, and sometimes outright pathology. For example, the kindergarten child who obsessively erases a letter of the alphabet is not making a mistake, but neither is he progressing to writing. If he continues to apply this schema, he will be at risk for mood disorders associated with poor self-esteem.

Children are particularly predisposed to perfectionism when they have had excessively critical parents or have been forced to make responsible choices at an early age. As one develops into adulthood, the consequences to body and mind can be profound. Numerous studies have found perfectionistic thinking to underlie teenage anorexic syndrome and suicide, and mood disorders at all ages.

An emotional downside to perfectionist thinking is that one rarely experiences satisfaction or peace of mind. One's standards of success are set with ideal precision in mind. Anything short of the goal is a failure, but achieving a goal means that one's criteria for success had been set too low and must now be adjusted upward. For example, a recent study of doctoral-level clinical psychologists found that personal satisfaction with their practice was inversely correlated with both their tendency to perfectionism and their tolerance for ambiguity.[1]

Having perfectionistic guidelines rarely points to one's eventual mastery of a field. Perfectionistic thinking, to the extent that it demands a certain outcome, prevents people from mastering a subject by inhibiting them from attempting new levels of performance or exploring new domains. The apprehensiveness associated with perfectionism can produce anything from stage fright to paralysis of the will. An ice skating coach pointed out to me that one can spot the best skaters by the fact that they fall to the ice more often. The poorer skaters are so afraid of falling that they cease to make progress. Fear of failure also prevents someone who has had success in one discipline from attempting something new. This has a crippling effect on the creative process, since those who leave their mark on a discipline often were initially trained in a different field.

> *Perfectionistic thinking, to the extent that it demands a certain outcome, prevents people from mastering a subject by inhibiting them from attempting new levels of performance or exploring new domains.*

Some perfectionists can push past their apprehension and thereby achieve formal recognition, or, in school, produce superior grades and standardized test scores. This is accomplished, in part, by assuming the judge's or teacher's values and criteria for success. Of course this fails to satisfy, since the perfectionist who successfully accommodates his instructor immediately realizes the inferiority of the test criteria relative to his own, unattainable, standards. It is for this reason that individuals who are viewed by society's standards as very successful, and are most appreciated by their teachers and judges, often view themselves as imposters. Most "imposters" believe that they can achieve the ultimate criteria of perfection if they try hard enough, while a fortunate few are able to work themselves free.

In contrast to the criteria-oriented perfectionist, the student who asks too many questions, or is inclined to more divergent thinking, or is passionate for areas not covered on the SAT, typically receives inconsistent marks, and is considered by his instructor as "reluctant" or "challenging."[2] For this individual to excel, he must believe in himself enough to risk failing, and enjoy the process enough to right himself on falling.

Heroism involves launching one's self toward the horizon, knowing not what lies beyond, but only that the process will bring change. The criteria-oriented perfectionist will freeze with indecision since he cannot know for certain the consequence of any particular course of action. And though he may follow another's map, he harbors the suspicion that another, superior, path exists. By contrast, the creative individual with a dream of perfection faces the void knowing that he can create a path for himself and those who may follow.

While there is no shortage of perfectionists (several of my patients have been lobbying for a place in this chapter), it is a rarity to find a perfectionist who manages to be productive over an extended period. Leni Riefenstahl (1902 – 2003) was a creative perfectionist for at least eighty-five years, starting with dance and successively redirecting her energies to acting, filmmaking, and still photography.

Leni Riefenstahl exhibited perfectionist thinking from her earliest memory of insisting that her father tell her exactly how many stars there were in the sky. Throughout her life, she had little patience for those not sharing her need for precision and positivistic philosophy.

In her teenage years, Leni engaged in a power struggle with her father over her studying dance. Her father finally conceded, saying, "I am willing to consent to your training as a dancer. Personally, I am convinced that you have little talent, and will never be more than mediocre." In some ways this blistering judgment echoes the voice of Charles Darwin's father, who sent his son off on the *Beagle* voyage with the comment: "I always knew you would never be good for anything but rat catching." Charles answered his father by spending the next twenty years of his life quietly striving to perfect his theories. Leni, on hearing her father's sentiments, set the highest possible standards for herself, endlessly practicing dance to prove her father wrong. Even after leaving dance as a career, Leni strove so as to never look weak.

Her drive to achieve kept her very much present-centered, with little time to reflect on the course of her life. Leni begins her 1987 autobiography saying, "It is not easy for me to leave the present behind and to immerse myself in the past in order to understand my life in all its strangeness. I have…like the waves of the ocean, never known rest."[3] She always had the ability to concentrate her energies on the creative project at hand, obtaining rest only from the physical collapse that inevitably would accompany a project's completion.

Every detail of a Riefenstahl creation bears the mark of a critical eye. In 1925, Leni was acting in a film, *The Holy Mountain*, written expressly for her, during which time she learned essentials of film direction. An insight that stayed with her was that "everything has to be equally well photographed: people, animals, clouds, water, ice. Every single shot…had to be above mere mediocrity."

In 1930, Leni invested all of her resources in producing *The Blue Light*, a fantasy set in a secluded mountain village, based on images she had played with since fifteen. Leni wrote, starred in, and directed the film. On reviewing the rushes, Leni was outraged that the editor had "mutilated" her film. In order to gain quality control over the creative product, she began her career as a film editor, and produced the most critically acclaimed German film of 1932.

> In order to salvage my film, I began editing it from scratch. From the thousands of tiny snippets, which I had to splice back together, I gradually wove a real film, which became more visible from week to week. At last the legend of *The Blue Light*, which had been a dream just one year earlier, lay before me: completed.
>
> — *Leni Riefenstahl: A Memoir*

The successful completion of *The Blue Light* was pivotal in Leni's life "because Hitler was so fascinated by the film that he insisted I make a documentary…*Triumph of the Will*." She began lengthy negotiations with Hitler, who eventually conceded to her complete artistic control over filming the National Socialist Party Rally of 1934.

It should not be surprising that Leni personally managed every aspect of the film's production. In order to complete the film and sound editing on schedule, Leni and her crew worked eighteen or nineteen hours a day, making sure that each frame was perfect. A march had been written especially for one segment of the film, and was to be recorded by an eighty-piece orchestra. Of course, neither the orchestra conductor nor the composer was adequate to the task of conducting the march, leaving Leni to conduct the music herself! She was able to keep herself going through the film's completion, collapsing at the screening and requiring five weeks rest before starting her next project.

Often one's personal reflections are heard in someone else's words. Leni recounts a meeting with Adolf Hitler in which she shared her apprehensions about documenting the 1936 Olympic Games to her standards. She recalls Hitler advising her: "You have to have a lot more self-confidence. What you do will be valuable, even if it remains incomplete in your eyes. Who else but you should make an Olympic film?" To me, the above voice sounds more like Leni Riefenstahl than Hitler. Perhaps she has unconsciously reconstructed her account so as to describe, through the most tyrannical voice possible, the inadequacy felt by all perfectionists. She would have dismissed anyone other than the Führer telling her that her work was valuable even if it failed to meet her own criteria.

The war years shattered Leni's social world and shook her out of her political naiveté. In 1940, one of her film projects was interrupted because of the war effort; Leni's nerves were shaken and she developed periodic colicky pains associated with cystitis. In July of 1944, Germany was collapsing both internally and from the Allied bombing runs each afternoon. Leni's father died and her brother was killed on the Russian front within days of each other. The stress, along with a diet of cheap carbohydrates, aggravated her chronic cystitis. The pain increased in severity over the next six years to the point of making walking difficult. She recovered as she entertained ideas for new films, along with an improved diet and a dose of antibiotics.

In the post-war years, Leni was ostracized from much of the artistic community that once had adored her. From 1950 to 1975 she initiated fourteen independent film projects, gaining physical strength from the promise of each. Unfortunately, each project was eventually aborted, primarily because of financial backers having second thoughts about hiring "Hitler's propagandist." Undaunted, Leni, dedicated herself to portrait and documentary photography, first in Africa and later in the oceans.

Leni always had a quality that was often self-limiting in perfectionists, namely, admitting into her world no shades of gray. For example, she would contract a film project only if she was assured complete control. This undoubtedly limited her artistic opportunities. Or consider how each of the romantic relationships she discusses was immediately and irrevocably terminated by her on finding that her partner had taken up with another, more available, woman. There was no discussion, working through, or consideration of her own role in the breach of confidence.

Of course, all-or-nothing thinking can also be a source of strength. For example, Leni had a serious car accident that forced her into hospital for several weeks, during which time she reflected on her "unbearable struggle for sheer existence" and became addicted to morphine prescribed to alleviate pain. "During those weeks in the hospital, the darkest in my life, I vegetated without a single shred of hope." On learning that she had unwittingly become addicted, Leni decided she had had enough of this and, in a move reminiscent of Norman Cousins', checked herself out of the hospital. Rather than following the doctor's regime of weaning off the morphine gradually, she immediately stomped on the ampules, and bore two weeks of torturous withdrawals.

Leni exhibited the best qualities of the creative perfectionist: concentrating her attention on the project of the moment, fighting to avoid compromising her criteria for perfection, believing in her vision enough to take risks, and recreating herself when needed. Physically, she had amazing recuperative powers that allowed her to repeatedly drive to the edge of exhaustion and then become energized by the thought of the next project. At the age of ninety-eight she completed her ninth book of photographs, and at ninety-nine, a feature length art film photographed underwater, of course by Leni herself.

Sister Agnes

The notion that there exists an expert physician who can size up your approaching death is recent in Western culture. Prior to the seventeenth century, each individual was considered the leading authority on his or her own state of health. If you determined that you were ill, you might consult someone for theological advice or a folk remedy, or, if you could afford it, hire someone knowledgeable in the healing arts whose payment was contingent upon your being cured. And if you sensed that your "days were numbered," you would alert every significant person in your life (including your physician) and put your affairs in order.

There are hints, which no one enjoys looking at, that the end of life is stealthily approaching. The number of natural teeth in our mouths steadily decreases, an increasing number of our classmates appear in the obituaries, and time seems to be going by faster with each year. What we may call an "entropic" paradigm is represented by the slogan, "Life sucks and you die." It is also the paradigm most representative of Chinese medicine, which asserts that we are born with a certain amount of Qi and then use it up until we are dead.

On another hand, the majority of folks try not to look at the signs of degeneration. There is the hope that we can continue with our lives indefinitely if only "someone" could find the secret elixir. Such dreams are encouraged by the scientific study of longevity as well as by quacks playing off our fears. When fearful, we are most likely to look to others for a solution.

Yet another paradigm views our search for solutions external to our own behavior as the primary cause for ill health and progressive degeneration. According to Ayurveda, we are born with a certain amount of *Ojas* (*Qi*). Subsequently, each of our thoughts, words and actions either adds to or subtracts from our reservoir of *Ojas*. This theory imbues a feeling of great responsibility for one's own health. However, maintaining awareness of one's responsibility takes great discipline when it is ever so much easier to worry about that tomorrow.

Coming face-to-face with mortality can make your complacency go flush. Until you do, there always seems to be time to get around to making changes. Certain individuals will die much faster than even their doctors expect when they hear the pronouncement of their coming demise. Others take the authoritative voice as a challenge. Of this latter group, some will step up their efforts to find "the perfect" treatment or doctor, while a few will look to change their lives.

Agnes at the age of sixty-eight had been diagnosed with ovarian cancer, which has a poor prognosis because it is often detected in an advanced stage. It is typically estrogen-driven, making the greatest risk factor the number of years spent producing estrogen. Nuns who entered service early in life, as had Agnes, are at increased risk because they have had no respite, by way of pregnancy, from estrogen production.

A few months after her first course of chemotherapy, cancerous cells had infiltrated to the liver and lungs, and the MRI showed lesions throughout her body. Her CA125 blood test (a measure of epithelial growth) was over 300, when we like to see it close to 1. Since there is no viable conventional therapy for generalized metastasis, the hospital chief of staff had referred Agnes to me.

She walked into my office with a purposeful step, appearing physically vital despite the headscarf, and showing no signs of accepting the dire prognostications from her various internists and oncologists. At the beginning of our conversation, Agnes described herself, in no uncertain terms, as a perfectionist. She elaborated that she would always persevere until something was done "right" (i.e., relative to her high standards). She was rarely, if ever, satisfied by the results, feeling that her projects were never really completed. She dealt with this feeling of incompleteness by always having new projects on which to work.

Many cancer patients refuse to change their lives in the face of their diagnosis, wanting symptomatic treatment to allow them to finish their work. Fortunately, Agnes is definitely not the "I can't stop" kind of person. I recall my astonishment at Agnes' determination to discover a more perfect self. On receiving confirmation of her cancer, she resigned as a school administrator and head of a non-profit board, not to ready herself for death but to redirect her energies to healing.

There was an obvious discrepancy between Agnes' vitality and her advanced metastatic disease that was perhaps twenty years in the making. It was apparent to both of us that she must have tuned out warning signs for many years for cancer cells to spread across her body unnoticed.

We discussed the basic physiology of cancer, including mechanisms the body uses to manage cancer on a daily basis. Hearing this, Agnes reflected that she felt that her body had failed her again.

"I've always been doing battle with my body. It gets in the way or lets me down when I need to do something important."

"Agnes, we're a cooperative effort between the body, mind, and spirit. Our bodies have ways of getting our attention when we neglect them. The good news is that you're listening and your body still has the strength to respond."

We then discussed those foods known to fight cancer. The foods on the "avoid" list are problematic because they either (a) contain animal or synthetic estrogens (hormone-fed meat and dairy), (b) fuel cancer cell growth (high glycemic foods, peanut lectin, linoleic acid), (c) are rich sources of the amino acids methionine or phenylalanine, or (d) are acidifying.

The "Good to Eat" list contains foods shown in large epidemiological studies or well-controlled clinical trials to help prevent or fight cancer. For the purposes of fighting generalized metastasis, it is essential to counter the acidosis that develops within and between cells. Acidosis arises as a consequence of the immune system or

The Anti-Cancer Diet

Foods to Avoid:

Red meat, hormone-fed meat or dairy, alcohol (occasional red wine is OK), white sugar, white flour, coffee, sunflower seeds, anise, hops, peanuts, peanut oil, corn oil, chlorinated water. Soybean or safflower oils are probably OK so long as they are fresh and used to lightly cook vegetables.

Generally Supportive Foods:

Fresh, vine-ripened, colorful fruits and vegetables, yams, sweet potatoes, cooked tomatoes, whole oats, brown rice, milk, lemon/lime, pure spring water.

Good To Eat:

Spinach, broccoli, artichokes, sunchokes, shitake mushrooms.

Lentils, miso, broadbeans (fava), garbanzo beans.

Green tea, oolong with chrysanthemum tea, grapefruit water.

Grapefruit (except during chemotherapy), berries (esp. blueberries), figs, black currents, amalki, apricots, almonds.

Extra-virgin olive oil, grapeseed oil, wheat germ oil, coconut milk, clarified butter.

Jerusalem artichoke flour.

Yoghurt, cottage cheese.

Seafood (esp. sardines), duck, goose, turtle, escargot!

Ginger, turmeric, onion, rosemary, lavender.

Figure 6.1. The Anti-Cancer Diet

chemotherapy killing cancer cells. A high acid environment makes healthy cells more vulnerable to infiltration; it is also responsible for much of the patient's discomfort. Accordingly, most of the recommended foods promote an alkaline environment.

Agnes immediately renounced her morning coffee for green tea. Numerous studies have found green tea to slow down the progress of reproductive cancers by protecting healthy cells and increasing alkalinity.

Just as corn and peanut oils facilitate the spread of cancer, certain foods (e.g., extra-virgin olive, fish, escargot) have oils and lectins that protect the intercellular space. Both shitake and maitake mushrooms have lectins that inhibit metastasis, though only shitake are sold as a food in the U.S.. Agnes began to supplement her diet with a standardized liquid extract of maitake mushrooms.

Agnes recognized the importance of substituting fish, which is pH neutral, for red meat, which is highly acidic. Besides the benefits of being a non-acidic protein source, fish oil is anti-inflammatory and, like other short-chained fatty acids, acts as support for the immune system. There is laboratory, animal, and human clinical evidence that fish oil and vitamin E are effective in treating generalized metastasis. For example, Gogos, et al (1998), in the journal *Cancer*, gave patients either a placebo or 200 mg of vitamin E plus 18 grams of fish oil. Over the following months, the treatment group had a significant increase in immune T-helper cells, along with significantly greater rates of survival.[4] Agnes would supplement with 800 IU of vitamin E and, when not eating fish, take fish oil in capsules with meals.

Agnes was suffering from anxiety that kept her awake at night. Restless, she would get up and walk about her house. The anxiety was probably caused by two factors. Psychologically, Agnes was stressed by having to confront her mortality. This can be as big an issue for someone leading a monastic life as for anyone else. It was a particularly difficult problem for Agnes since she was accustomed to calculating the consequences of an action in advance, and now it appeared that her life was no longer in her own hands.

There was also a biochemical cause of Agnes' anxiety. Her body undoubtedly, had redirected its stores of melatonin to fighting cancer and away from its function of helping nightly sleep. After vitamin D3, the body's most important cancer fighter is melatonin, a hormone produced by the pineal gland (located near the optic nerve and between the limbic system and the brain stem). Melatonin is produced in response to sunlight stimulating the optic nerve, and stored for nighttime use twelve to thirteen hours later.

Melatonin serves as a hormone, a neurotransmitter, a brain antioxidant, an immune stimulant, and a cancer cell anti-proliferative. As a neurotransmitter, melatonin helps us sleep. As an immune stimulant, it increases the release of interleukin-2.[5] As an antioxidant, it cleans up hydroxyl radicals known to cause cancer.[6] And melatonin acts as an anti-proliferative by promoting connexin-32[7] and inhibiting the metabolizing of linoleic acid uptake.[8] Connexin-32 is a chemical found between cells that promotes communication between adjacent cells. Melatonin stimulates production of connexin-32, thereby helping the body to maintain regulatory control over healthy cells. By inhibiting the metabolizing of linoleic acid, melatonin denies cancer cells access to one of their favorite fuels. (Since corn oil and flaxseed oil are rich sources of linoleic acid, they are on the "Foods to Avoid" list.)

Given all the various physiologic pathways by which the body uses melatonin, it is not surprising to find it where the body is doing battle with cancer. In fact, high concentrations of melatonin have been found in breast cancer tissue: three orders of magnitude higher than that present in blood. Maestroni (1999) found that melatonin concentration in breast tissue correlates positively with a generally good prognosis as well as prognostic markers such as estrogen-receptor status.[9]

A number of studies have found clinical benefit in the treatment of all types of cancer from melatonin in potencies ranging from 20 to 40 mg. These amounts are much higher than our bodies typically produce, and might, eventually, inhibit the natural production of melatonin. Accordingly, I recommended to Agnes that she get sunlight exposure in the morning, sleep in a totally dark room at night, and supplement before bed with only that amount of melatonin needed to sleep easily without feeling groggy in the morning. While most individuals with a sleep disturbance find 1 to 3 mg of melatonin sufficient, Agnes was just able to get to sleep with 6 mg of melatonin and a homeopathic remedy that fit her restless perfectionism.

Two of the three homeopathic portraits which exhibit perfectionist tendencies are also prominent remedies to treat cancer. I decided to probe a little more into the nature of Agnes' self-proclaimed perfectionism. She believed that her perfectionism was deep rooted. Growing up, her mother had enforced an ever-growing list of "shoulds" for her to follow. The primary "should" was that she should know what to do without asking. This has the effect of making the child incorporate within her own psychological structures the will of the parent.

At the same time, it had been made painfully clear that her mother was disappointed in Agnes in a way that could never be satisfied. A year before Agnes was born, her mother's first son had died, and she periodically reminded Agnes of her disappointment at seeing a girl. A couple of years after Agnes' birth, another boy was born, and her earliest memories are of being dressed up in matching clothes with her little brother.

At age seventeen, Agnes brought to the novitiate a dogged determination to make things just right. Accordingly, she was assigned jobs that required a will to perfection. For example, she spent years sewing veils by hand. Each "gimp" in the front had nine pleats, and if the warp and woof were not lined up perfectly, she would start over.

Later, Agnes served in the Watts area of Los Angeles, functioning as principal, secretary, treasurer, a teacher and "the mother of the house." She understood that perfectionism could inhibit learning in her school children, and implemented measures to help prevent it. For example, her students were given pencils without erasers, and instructed to leave mistakes with a line drawn through them, followed by the correctly spelled word.

Agnes has always been aware of her perfectionism as well as a compulsion to make things orderly. In order to avoid being limited by these tendencies, she trained herself to not see disorder. For example, apprehensive that a superior might ask for a racial count in her school, she made a point of not knowing how many black children there were. Or, knowing that she might be unable to resist organizing her housemate's side of the office, Agnes erected a folding screen so as to obstruct her view.

I gave Agnes homeopathic *Arsenicum*, to be taken when feeling restless. Individuals who respond favorably to *Arsenicum* tend to be anxious, restless perfectionists who are easily disturbed by disorder or the threat of disorder. They have a fear of becoming too disabled to function perfectly, while simultaneously believing that, "It's a dangerous world for which you cannot be too prepared." They can become so anguished by these thoughts that they start pacing or are driven out of bed to walk throughout the house. I once had a patient in the midst of an asthmatic attack who started pacing in my office while straightening pictures on the walls! A single dose of *Arsenicum* allowed her to lie down and take a restful nap. I instructed Agnes that she should use the drug sparingly since in homeopathy "less is often more."

Our next consultation was four weeks later. On the positive side, she had found the *Arsenicum* to calm her, and, in conjunction with the melatonin, was able to sleep. However, Agnes' CA125 score was still in the 300s, and her physicians held little hope for her recovery. She had been unable to screen out the negative prognosis and was feeling lost.

At this point, I realized that I had no magic bullets to fix Agnes. However, there are times when the patient's body dramatically comes back on line. I felt that for Agnes the spiritual domain held the most promise to wake her body's healing power, especially in the context of her willingness to renounce jobs that were draining her. Moreover, the feeling of "being at wit's end" might open her to discovering a healthier self.

I asked her when she felt most like herself, and she responded that she used to love to pray. Cautiously, I asked Agnes, "Do you pray now?"

She responded matter-of-factly, "As a young nun I prayed twice a day, but I have had little time for it in the past twenty years or so."

"It sounds like you must have enjoyed it?"

"It was my reason for being a nun, but the monastic life is also filled with service and responsibility."

Whenever hearing "It was my reason for being, but…" it strikes me that we are dealing with a critical decision turned awry, or, more fundamentally, the will turned against itself. I took a deep breath and proceeded to discuss a traditional Tibetan prayer.

"There is a Tibetan prayer or meditation called *Tong-Len*, two words meaning receiving and giving. It is used to bring peace to yourself and your world." Agnes appeared interested, so I continued. "It is in some ways just the reverse from Western imagery techniques in which you "breathe in the good air and blow out the bad." Instead, on the in-breath you allow the suffering about you to enter, you hold the breath for a moment feeling that suffering, and then on the out-breath you feel a wave of compassion going to that same place."

Agnes asked me if *Tong-Len* could be directed toward one's own body. She had "always felt that she was doing battle with it" and now felt that it was time to make peace. I explained that this is considered the highest form of Tibetan Ayurvedic medicine used to heal the body.

When I saw Agnes the following month, she was exuding a sense of ease and accomplishment. Without a word, she presented her laboratory reports. Her CA125 had plummeted from 300 to 9, and her MRIs showed no evidence of lesions where they had previously existed in countless abundance. The blood and imaging analyses had been reconfirmed, both finding that "there is no evidence of cancer."

I have continued to consult with Agnes on a regular basis for the past five years. A year ago, her CA125 score climbed up to 30, causing some consternation in both of us. We decided to review the stressors in Agnes' life, and it became apparent that in her recovery years she had gradually taken on more and more responsibility. An administrator can ask nothing more than to have a perfectionist working for him, and so Agnes was much sought after in her religious community. She was now teaching specialized classes to novices and was serving on various committees.

Agnes interpreted her elevated cancer marker as an outcome of stress. Once again, she chose to let go of activities feeding on her perfectionist drive, turning down new assignments and phasing out commitments that pulled her this way and that. She returned to her daily practice of *Tong-Len*. Within a matter of weeks, Agnes' CA125 dropped, this time to 13.

Reflecting on her ability to control the rate at which her body produces new cancer cells has inspired Agnes to share her personal experiences with cancer patients. The basic message is that your body and mind, and what you choose to do with them, can be the cause of illness or the most powerful medicine.

Agnes' case has affected me deeply. It is one thing to know that oncology studies indicate that psychological counseling yields the most positive results of any therapy; it is far more impressive to see your patient eliminate cancer by making fundamental changes in her life.

Until a perfectionist is truly at wit's end, he or she is more likely to merely try harder than to change course in life.

It is so rare for someone to make a fundamental change in his or her life that it seems miraculous when they do. For perfectionists, a serious illness presents a complex problem that requires their full attention as they make a plan and organize the best possible team of specialists. So long as they can focus on the details, they are not motivated to scrutinize the role their mode of living may be playing in perpetuating the illness.

Until a perfectionist is truly at wit's end, he or she is more likely to merely try harder than to change course in life. Both Leni Riefenstahl and Agnes reinvented their relationship to the world only after finding themselves stranded where effort and expertise failed to light a path to satisfaction. Leni gave up her motion picture career and took up portrait and documentary photography and social causes (e.g., the abolition of African slave trade). Agnes quit administrative responsibilities, rediscovered prayer, and began conducting cancer support groups.

St. John of the Cross argued that "the dark night of the soul" is necessary for spiritual development. Having hit bottom, one is not distracted by desires to attain perfection in either this world or the next, or fears of losing one's possessions or social support. Without hopes and fears, what remains in one's consciousness clearly lights a new way. This may be experienced as love or redemption, or a new domain for creative expression.

Tarique

It is debilitating for an artist to be a perfectionist. An empty canvas or page can be frightening, tempting him or her to delay the first brush- or keystroke until everything is perfectly in order. Even after stocking one's studio with the best equipment, it is impossible to create something new if you are waiting for assurances about the creative product's eventual public reception. An even more profound problem, particularly for the creation of representational art, is capturing the beauty of a scene without forfeiting its imperfections. Incorporating real-world irregularities within a work of art communicates to the viewing audience the artist's chiseled vision of the moment. Armed with the necessary technical skills, a creative artist struggles to grasp the moment without being distracted by the vision of perfection and the temptation to peek at the finished product.

Tarique is a twenty-two-year-old with an engaging, though serious, countenance, and with features verging on pretty. Only after he described his chief complaint as exfoliative cheilitis, did I notice that his lips were somewhat swollen and peeling. Two years ago, Tarique had gone to his physician with severe sunburn on his neck, face and lips, for which he was given a topical cortisone cream. His lips peeled and never recovered, despite topical and systemic steroids to reduce the inflammation, and an interventionist therapy in which the top layer of cells were chemically removed. Despite his best efforts, the condition would resurface every few days, and had made him very self-conscious of his appearance.

I checked his mouth for signs of a yeast infection, but he was clear. Tarique had discovered methods that helped a little. By avoiding toothpastes with carvone or other additives that can elicit a chemical reaction, the intensity of the inflammation could be lessened; avoiding alcohol, meat, or sun exposure to his lips seemed to delay the onset of lesions. Tarique would always carry a straw with him in case he needed a drink, thereby protecting his lips from getting wet.

I asked Tarique what *he* thought was the cause of the chronic cheilitis, and, without hesitation, he replied "stress and fatigue." The stress was related to a difficult home situation and frustration about not being able to dedicate himself to his love of photography.

He had lost twenty-five pounds since becoming ill, and was now a gaunt 120 pounds. A blood test showed abnormally low levels of cortisol, an adrenal hormone responsible for managing inflammation and the rise and fall of energy throughout the day. Tarique may have fallen victim to the allopathic practice of supplementing with synthetic cortisone (e.g., prednisone), which eventually gives the unintended message to the body that it need not produce its own cortisone.

Like many individuals suffering from adrenal fatigue and its related depression, Tarique had low blood pressure that would become even lower when standing. It went from 90/60 sitting, to 80/55 standing. Upon standing, blood pressure, as measured at the arm, always drops briefly as blood rushes to the feet. But the drop typically cannot be measured, because a healthy body quickly redirects blood upward. In so-called orthostatic hypotension, the brain, adrenals and circulatory systems fail to compensate for this drop, making one feel lightheaded and dizzy.

I recommended that Tarique add salt to his diet (he had eliminated it "for health reasons") to help his body hold moisture and increase blood volume. I also recommended that he start each morning by massaging the soles of his feet, moving from the heel up to a typically tender spot known in Chinese medicine as *Kidney One* or *Gushing Spring*. This is the beginning of the kidney meridian, and is thought to be responsible for dispersing energy and fluid throughout the body.

The standard practice in conventional medical treatment of cheilitis is to use either immune suppression (steroids) or immune stimulation (imiquimod). In fact, cheilitis may be a condition in which both approaches are necessary: suppression of inflammatory pathways of the immune system along with stimulation of interferon. There is evidence that licorice extract is both anti-inflammatory and an interferon booster, besides providing support to weary adrenals. Licorice, when taken on a daily basis, also increases blood pressure by affecting the kidneys and adrenals. Accordingly, I recommended that Tarique take licorice capsules and apply licorice ointment to his lips at night. He was also prescribed an encapsulated formula for adrenal support, with licorice extract, vitamin C, pantothenic acid, and adrenal extract.

As far as diet was concerned, I cautioned Tarique about consuming cheap carbohydrates since they tend to depress the immune system. These are the typically white foods that people find comforting, such as table sugar, white bread, and white potatoes. Rather, I recommended good oils, especially that from coconut milk because of its ability to support the immune system while decreasing inflammation.

A month later, Tarique and I met again. His lips were puffy but not peeling and his energy was "maybe a little better." His blood pressure was 95/60 sitting, decreasing only moderately to 90/55 upon standing.

I asked him to describe his family life since he had indicated that this was a cause of health-compromising stress. Tarique's family had moved from Nairobi to Austria when he was eight and then to the U.S. when he was ten. Settling into California, his parents soon divorced and he lost touch with his father. Tarique's mother was "a very successful exotic dancer" in a local nightclub. He remembers, as a twelve year old, observing his mother carefully selecting breast implants that would perfectly complement the rest of her body. As a teenager, he had taken a lurid portrait of his mother "drenched in fake sweat."

Tarique's home always had buffed young men plying for his mother's favor. Drug use in the house steadily increased over the years, leaving Tarique to fend for himself while keeping a watchful eye on his mother. Tarique's maternal grandmother was an artist in Vienna, and had periodically "rescued" the family with money. This source of support had disappeared when it became apparent that the money was not supporting nutrition and "artistic development." The loss of financial support posed real problems, but it also served to motivate Tarique to change his living accommodations.

Since I had last seen Tarique, he had decided that he could no longer be responsible for what might happen to his mother. He had left home, and was living out of his car and eating handouts from restaurants. He was reluctant to look for work because of his appearance, and his depressed energy level, and because it might mean forsaking his artistic aspirations. I suggested that we focus first on getting him a place to eat and sleep. I offered him a bottle of *chyvanprash* (an Ayurvedic chutney rich in essential fatty acids, vitamins and balancing herbs). Tarique made a few telephone calls and found people willing to offer room and board in return for help around the house. We would discuss his creative work when he was better fed.

At our next meeting, two weeks later, Tarique obviously had more vitality, and we discussed his photography. He had an eye for abstracting the geometrical shapes of common objects, bringing that shape to the fore in the photo. I was particularly impressed by his black and white close-ups of faces.

Tarique had not taken photos for nearly a year because he could not arrange the perfect environment for it. Without his own home, he had no studio where he could control lighting and work uninterrupted. Without an income, he lacked the funds to purchase film, filters, and supplies for film developing. Even if the technical support was there, he lacked sufficient energy to see a project through to its completion. And, now that he had not produced anything in so long, he doubted that there would be an audience for his pictures.

In fact, it seemed to Tarique that perhaps he had been fooling everyone in regard to his abilities.

We discussed how insisting on perfect circumstances and a receptive audience before engaging a project prevents the creation of new ideas, or, at the very least, deprives one of satisfaction. Creative inspiration may be defined as the integration of ideas drawn from disparate domains, e.g., Darwin's integration of the political economics' concept of competition within his theory of evolution of species by natural selection. Our ability to create requires appreciation for an unresolved situation while we consider disparate problem-domains rich with possibilities. In fact, the longer we endure the tension of an ambiguous situation before projecting the best outcome, the greater the opportunity to discover new ways of combining existing ideas. It is the appreciation for ambiguity that most clearly distinguishes between the unrequited perfectionist and the perfectionist who enjoys the creative process.

Tarique was feeling so torn between competing possibilities that he was at wit's end as to how to proceed. He asked, "How do you know which is the best thing to do?" The search for the *best* path is indicative of perfectionism and, when facing competing voices, can lock one into a cycle of obsessive thinking.

"Tarique, it sounds like you are hearing lots of opinions as to what you should do, some coming from people around you, other voices coming from yourself. What, exactly, are the voices saying?"

"Most of the time I hear 'You can't do it.' You know, all the reasons why I can't do my photography. Other times, I think how good it would be to have an easy life, eventually get a job, a family, and the things of the world."

"Do you really think that you *can't* do your photography if that is what you choose to do? It sounds to me as though you, or people that you are listening to, do not value a creative pursuit as much as a life in the world. Maybe struggling to become a photographer is something that you *shouldn't* do?"

"My grandmother says that I can do it, but my mother and friends tell me that my head is in the clouds. I don't know what I think."

I explained to Tarique that *not knowing* can be a blessed place in the creative process, but only so long as he can live with the uncertainty. Creative insight typically follows a period of so-called "incubation" when various possibilities are being quietly observed and considered. The model is that of a fertile egg, in which a great deal of development is happening out of sight until the chick suddenly breaks from its shell. Unlike the chick, humans can choose to foster and endure their own process of incubation.

I asked Tarique if he believed that those who spoke of the superiority of worldly comforts really were living an easy and happy life. The answer came quickly: "They're older and speak with confidence, but their faces show fear."

"Tarique, whenever I hear voices calling for me to get my head out of the clouds, I remember a beautiful summer day I spent hiking in Vancouver. My lady friend and I had taken the ski lift up Grouse Mountain and had hiked into the woods. She decided to stay at an overlook while I hiked on. Unfortunately, we had not brought water or food and, in the thin air, I had underestimated the distance to the next peak. Six hours later, I was crossing a snow bridge, a narrow ledge of snow filling the area between mountain peaks and sloping precipitously to either side for a depth of approximately a kilometer. Half way across, I suffered total fatigue. My legs began to shake and I felt no physical or mental strength to carry on. At this point, I heard the most comforting voice imaginable speaking to me from the bottom of the snow bridge, 'You can rest down here,' the compelling nature of that Siren-like voice scared the hell out of me. My adrenals kicked in and I made it across the bridge and back to my friend just as darkness fell."

Tarique summarized the moral of the story. "Those who promise us comfort might just be trying to pull us down to their level. Also, stay the course and don't forget to bring food and water!"

I asked Tarique how his cheilitis had changed his life. As a child and teenager, he had been "told by everyone how beautiful or perfect" he looked. Being the center of attention had given him a sense of social confidence, though it reinforced a sense of skepticism about people's judgment. The exfoliating lips left him with an obvious imperfection. Those who had doted on him turned their attentions to his mother, making him more of an observer. Ever since, he has been hiding his face from public scrutiny. His interests had turned to photography and spiritual exercises such as yoga and meditation. He recognized that the cheilitis had served him well by motivating him to redirect his energy to his inner world and allowing him to see who were his true friends.

I probed further, and inquired if the cheilitis interfered with his developing romantic relationships. Tarique felt that he could not kiss a woman, and that, "No woman would give me a chance at a love relationship." We sat quietly for a moment with what had just been said. I was thinking about a female patient who had shown me a photo of herself taken some ten years earlier when she had been eighty pounds lighter and obviously proud of her physical beauty. She said that she had not trusted the advances of anyone looking at her and had knowingly gained the weight as her "insulation." Tarique interrupted my musings by commenting, "I've thought that maybe I'm hanging onto this disease as a way of protecting myself from anyone who is not interested in *me*."

I could no longer resist my psychological proclivities and asked if his mother was truly interested in him. Tarique allowed himself tears, and a moment later choked out, "She hasn't a clue who I am." I asked him if his mother loved him, and he replied that he felt she did in her own way.

I sensed that Tarique was now at a place in his life where his actions could make a difference in his health. "From what you've told me, hiding your face served to redirect your attention from outer to inner beauty, but I don't think it helps you any longer."

"It's not just that I was hiding my face; I've been hiding behind my face."

"But now there are people around you who respect you for your creative potential. So, it might be time to shed your skin and follow your heart." I further recommended that Tarique resume taking photographs, with special attention paid to facial expressions.

To help restore physical energy I recommended that Tarique practice each morning and evening a series of *Qi Gong* exercises. *Qi*

Tibetan Qi Gong

1.   Foot Massage. Rub each arch from back to front with circling hand movements, concentrating finger pressure on *Gushing Spring* (a typically tender point on the arch between big and second toes).

2.   (a) Turning. With knees slightly bent, arms loose, palms feel warmth radiating from the ground, take small steps in a clockwise direction (right arm moving backwards). As your speed increases allow your arms to rise slightly above the head; return to initial position as you slow down. Repeat, moving in a counter-clockwise direction, and, finally, clockwise again. Rest until breath and vision stabilizes.

(b) Rocking (Vata). On a rug or mat, sit with knees up; hands behind knees. On in-breath, rock backwards onto shoulders, and, breathing out, forward again. Do 7 times. Feel the stimulation along your spine.

3.   The Tibetan Crunch. Lie on your back on a rug or mat, arms at sides, palms down, feet together. On an in-breath, raise head and shoulders toward your chest while lowering back into the rug. Holding breath, raise legs as close to the vertical as possible. Relax out-breath while lowering legs and, then, upper torso to starting position. If hamstrings are too tight, bend knees as needed. Do 5 to 9 times.

4.   (a) Setting the Table (Pitta, Kapha). Sit upright with legs outstretched, feet 6 to 12 inches apart; hands at the hips, palms down, fingers pointing to your feet. On the in-breath, raise yourself onto your hands and feet, forming a *table*. This involves moving your torso upward while moving down over your feet. On the out-breath, slowly relax body to starting position. Do 5 to 9 times.

(b) Candlestick or Reversing Attitude (Vata). Lie on your back. Gently raise your body to the vertical, toes pointed, braising yourself on your shoulders and elbows with support from your hands against the lower back. Hold so long as you can breathe normally.

5.   The Spinal Cycle. Roll over and hold yourself up on hands and toes. Begin with arched head with pelvis just above the floor. On in-breath raise buttocks while lowering head so as to look between legs. On out-breath, return to starting position, raising eyes in the process. Until you develop strong enough muscles you may wish to support yourself on your knees rather than toes. Do 5 to 9 times.

Exercises 6-8 are best performed facing the sun. Stand with joints relaxed: allow the knees to bend forward, the pelvis and buttocks to relax downward, and shoulders to drop. Feel your hands "tingle" with Qi (energy).

6.   Crane goes Fishing. Stand with arms at sides, feet close together. Exhale completely by forcibly contracting abdominal muscles. Then glide your left foot forward while bending over at the waist, and bringing hands together in front of left foot. On in-breath, straighten your back while spreading your arms above your head at a 45-degree angle and raising your eyes: feel your lower back and chest fill with air, energy and joy (the Egyptian hieroglyph "Ka"). Holding breath, contract genital and perineum muscles, and hold for a few seconds. Exhale while gracefully returning to starting position. Repeat while advancing the right foot. Do the whole sequence 3 times.

Resume the basic standing position, with feet at least shoulder-width apart, joints relaxed. Rotate pelvis, allowing arms to loosely spin like a top. Slowly come back to center with palms feeling the warmth from your Dan Tian (the *lower burner*, in the middle of the body, below the naval).

7.   Bear Looking at the Moon. On the in-breath, rotate your upper body and head all the way to the left while allowing both arms to extend to the left, palms outwards as if framing the moon. Relax the breath out as you return to center, then repeat to the right. Do the whole sequence 3 times.

8.   Bathing the Face. Feel the warmth in your hands. Close your eyes and cover face with hands, fingers upwards. Slowly rub up and down over face and scalp several seconds; then gently cup your eyes until feeling relaxed and centered. Feel your lower back expand and contract with each breath.

Figure 6.2. Tibetan Qi Gong

Gong is an ancient Chinese, Tibetan, and Indian practice that resembles both yoga and *Tai Qi*. The particular exercises that I recommended are adaptations of the so-called "Five Tibetan Rites of Rejuvenation," supposedly brought from Tibet by a British colonel.[10] Many people have found that regular practice restores youthful appearance and vigor after they have suffered from adrenal fatigue. I have attempted to reconstruct the Ayurvedic nature of the original exercises. Individuals of different constitutional types perform different variations of the exercises. I have also modified the British version of these exercises so as to protect the exerciser from muscle strain. And, instead of performing an increasing number of repetitions, as in Western exercise, one performs the exercises slower and slower as his or her strength improves.

A month later, Tarique came into my office appearing taller and happier. I had not realized until then that he had stood somewhat stooped; only now was he standing relaxed with his spine in a straight line. It was also the first time that I noticed Tarique's smile; apparently, he had avoided smiling because it stretched his lips and aggravated the skin lesions.

He presented to me his portfolio of photos taken since we had last consulted. Tarique had asked his grandmother for money to cover the cost of the project, and she was happy to oblige. The series of twelve self-portraits were monochromatic (black and white with subtle gradations of red or blue, as was commonly produced in the 1940s). As I studied the photos, a theme emerged. The first in the series appeared mask-like, with expressive eyes (perhaps with a look of fear) peering out from behind the skin. But as we moved through the series, the face and eyes progressively represented an integrated expression of emotion. The final picture showed a handsome young man with a relaxed, toothy smile and glistening eyes.

CHAPTER SEVEN

Hubris

Patients often dismiss physicians as being *conceited*, while physicians refer to patients as *vain* and neurotic. Whether it is perception or actual behavior, we are dealing with a lack of understanding that has dire consequences to the healing process.

The word *conceit* denotes an obsessive appreciation of one's own worth, especially one's ability to grasp a situation. So long as we believe that we already know what is needed, we are blind to the uniqueness of a situation and not open to new perspectives. For example, a doctor looking to confirm a disease he sees quite often may overlook a fatal, though uncommon, disorder. *Vanity*, like the word *vanish*, comes from the Latin *vanitas*, meaning empty or valueless. It denotes inflated pride in oneself, especially in one's appearance. When attention is fixated on appearances, the perceived self (or ego) inflates, transporting the person even further from the depths of their psyche. Gradually, one loses touch and then sight with his or her psychological center. Like the Cheshire cat's smile in *Alice in Wonderland*, one is eventually left with nothing but a placid expression.

Consider the cancer patient consulting with his or her oncologist. Almost all patients are in a trance-like state with their lives on the line and hearing pronouncements from someone who has taken the mantle of authority. With the patient's attention fixed on the massive desk and white lab coat, the physician appears larger than life and his words are accepted literally and taken to heart. The following statements are taken from actual practice. "You have three to four months to live, so you'd better get your things in order." "If you do not take this chemotherapy, you will most likely die a painful death." Whether or not they are spoken with as much conceit as they sound, such pronouncements promote a superficial (vain) following of orders, and a belief that life is out of one's control; they are, therefore, detrimental to the patient's health.

Many patients falsely believe that it would be arrogant to ask the physician for more information or a human perspective on their condition. But, in fact, it is their due. Moreover, cancer patients who challenge their doctors live longer, even if their doctors are annoyed in the process! Fortunately, some physicians take the emotional risk of engaging with the patient. "I am here to support you as you fight this cancer." "I believe chemotherapy will be instrumental in helping you fight the disease. Take your time and tell me how or what you're feeling right now."

A sure sign that you are dealing with someone whose vanity has outstripped their sense of inner worth is when they display redundant or auxiliary monikers. People who identify themselves, for example, as Dr. So-And-So, BA, MS, PhD, MD, FAAP make us wonder why they are trying so hard to impress. Such vanity often appears on the physician's wall. One of my professors had hanging behind his desk fifteen diplomas and certificates, including his Boy Scout merit award!

Across languages, cultures, and human history, there have been an inordinate number of words and stories denoting the concept of pride and its dangers when taken to excess. Conventional wisdom within the disciplines of psychology and anthropology is that, wherever words persist that serve to discriminate numerous shades of meaning (e.g., types of "snow" to an Eskimo), we have a concept central to the survival and well being of that culture.

Of the nexus of words related to *pride*, relatively few have neutral or positive connotations. The word *pride* comes from the Latin *prodesse,* meaning to be virtuous. *Confidence* comes from the Latin *confidentia* meaning trust, though in contemporary times it may be used ironically as an adjective, e.g., "a confidence scheme." The Hebrew word *ratzon* denotes boundless confidence that is both divinely inspired and innocent of consequences. The biblical example is that of Adam in the radiant period of Paradise when he alone shared God's will or desire. The Yiddish *chutzpah* originally was synonymous with *effrontery* (meaning "putting forth the forehead" or shameless), *haughty* (Old French *haut* meaning high), and *insolent* (Latin *insolens* meaning "contrary to custom"). But today, international usage of *chutzpah* is synonymous with *audacity* (denoting actions that may have the positive virtue of being daring or bold).

The ancient Greeks used the term *hubris* to denote an outrageous violation of the order of things inevitably brought on by presuming power over heaven or nature. In the fifth century BCE, historian Herodotus recorded examples of hubris performed by Xerxes, the king of Persia. Xerxes ordered the construction of flax and papyrus bridges across the strait of Hellespont so his armies could cross and destroy the Greeks. But no sooner had the strait been bridged, than a great storm came on which cut apart and scattered their work. Xerxes flew into a rage at this. He commanded that the Hellespont be struck with three hundred strokes of the whip and that a pair of foot-chains be thrown into the sea. He also commanded the scourgers to speak outlandish and arrogant words: "You hateful water…Xerxes the king will pass over you, whether you wish it or not! It is fitting that no man offer you sacrifices for you're a muddy and salty river!"[1]

Undaunted, Xerxes ordered a bridge be built consisting of his naval vessels linked together. This "unnatural" conversion of sea into land was punished by the gods with the unexpected victory of the Greeks over the Persians.

Hubris and its consequences is the theme and moral of the oldest known stories. In an ancient tale from Acadia, Babylon, and Egypt, the god Set (etymologically related to "Satan") schemes to replace his brother, Osiris, by dismembering him and scattering his parts to the winds. The efforts of mother Isis and the faithful son Horus restore Osiris while exemplifying the path for human redemption.

The earliest known work of literature is the Sumerian *Epic of Gilgamesh*. Significantly, it is the story of a king's hubris, manifested by his destroying a pristine cedar forest and the hunting of creatures of heaven. The gods punish Gilgamesh by sending him a loving companion who mirrors him in all ways except possessing childlike innocence. The eventual death of his companion drives Gilgamesh to the depths of the underworld where he learns humility and the joys of the simple life.

Two other terms are typically listed as synonyms of hubris, though each reflects a different way in which excessive pride may unfold. The word *arrogance* is derived from the Latin *rogare* meaning to ask, and the Old French *rogue* meaning a beggar. As such, one who is arrogant asks for that which is not his due. Contrast this with the word *temerity*, which denotes foolhardy actions launched with ignorance of their consequences. It is derived from Latin *temere* meaning acting blindly; this, in turn, is derived from the Sanskrit *tamas,* meaning darkness, ignorance, inertia, and forgetfulness of one's real identity.

The classic tragedy *Oedipus Rex* illustrates both hubris and temerity. Oedipus is fated at birth to kill his father and marry his mother, and is unwittingly separated from his parents at birth. Learning of the prophecy, Oedipus is determined to take actions that will alter his destiny, thereby challenging the gods with an act of hubris. Of course, the more proactive, though blindly, he acts, the closer he comes to fulfilling the dreaded prophecy. For this, he is punished with the loss of his kingdom, witnessing the suicide of his wife-mother, and by imposing upon himself a cloak of perpetual darkness.

It appears that we are today as susceptible to hubris as people four thousand years ago. For example, a medical degree and a little fame give us someone who writes a book entitled *How to Know God*. I believe the most profitable question is whether hubris can serve our quest for health. The ancient philosophers and dramatists realized that it is our nature to challenge the fates and those influences that prevent fundamental change. Odysseus, on his circuitous route home, challenges the beasts of heaven, much as did Gilgamesh. But Odysseus, unlike Gilgamesh, experiences his personal torments as the price of independence rather than repentance for his transgressions. Odysseus has himself strapped to the ship's mast so as to hear the Siren's song and thereby witness himself resisting the voices of the gods. Throughout the voyage, he and his crew risk life, limb and sanity for the opportunity to make independent decisions.

The next time you see an advertisement or hear a personal claim that a physician is privy to a treatment that cures all or most people with a particular condition, escape with your life and money and seek a physician who will work with you.

Without some degree of hubris we may never stretch beyond our immediate grasp or think to carve out our own futures. Without some arrogance, we might not question whether we are due more than we get. Without temerity, we might not engage in a voyage of discovery without first knowing where it will lead.

There is hubris that is injurious and hubris that is essential to life. It is foolhardy for a patient to assume that he can learn medical science and how to apply it to himself. It is criminal (though rarely indicted) for a physician to intimate that he has a proprietary cure applicable to whomever has a particular diagnostic code and can foot the bill. The next time you see an advertisement or hear a personal claim that a physician is privy to a treatment that cures all or most people with a particular condition, escape with your life and money and seek a physician who will work with you. For example, my morning's electronic junk mail included an "infomercial" promising, "Your life will change forever. One free bottle…"

Good medicine always uses basic scientific knowledge to understand the uniqueness of the individual patient. Until recently, physicians were elite members of a secret society, selected for their intellect, character and social position, sworn to confidentiality, and learning the secrets of life and death. But, there are no medical secrets in today's egalitarian and Internet era. Everyone has access to the same, vast, amount of information, which makes it more important than ever to have research, interpersonal, and problem-solving skills with which to interpret and apply that knowledge. Using as much hubris as necessary, patients can exert a healthy sense of control over their lives by challenging their physicians to access their professional skills – both intellectual and psychological – and to apply them in a creative manner for the patient's benefit.

In today's medical education system, with its emphasis on emergency triage, normative evaluation, and standardized therapy, physicians are selected for their ability to quickly and accurately place a patient within a diagnostic category. Unfortunately, this ability can also prevent the physician from developing and accessing skills better suited for the treatment of chronically ill individuals.

One way to discover the hitch in someone's development is to ask what it is that they are good at. I worked with a psychologist who, without hesitation, answered, "I am a great listener. People come from all over to talk to me." After a moment of silence, she reflected that much of her personal stress came from the fact that she was reluctant to express her own opinion.

In general, we are most reluctant to give up those behaviors that have achieved success or those beliefs whose expression has gained approbation. While excessive pride obstructs change, a certain amount of confidence or even temerity is required to move beyond what is perceived to be your most positive virtue. I recall a middle-aged mechanic who had developed his career as an auto-repairman ever since his father complemented him on how good he was with his hands. He became depressed whenever he reflected that he had never truly felt like himself doing such work. With some encouragement to take a blind leap, he took an adult education course on designing clothes and is now enjoying a new career in fashion.

We all carry from our youth ghostly images that point a bony finger into the future. Such ghostly figures may have actually existed, but they are often shaped from our own hand and animated with every breath we give to them. In dozens of psychology experiments testing the limits of eyewitness testimony, subjects confidently identify a videotaped scene as having been *observed* when in fact the events had only been *thought* about. The more people replay their mental tapes of the event, the more confident they become of their false recognition.

In general, we are most reluctant to give up those behaviors that have achieved success or those beliefs whose expression has gained approbation.

Confidence, like hubris, can have either positive or negative consequences. Knowing that he had created a successful auto shop, the mechanic, who was previously discussed, had courage to venture into a new field. On the other hand, if fashion design had been merely the passion of the month, he would eventually face an even greater state of depression.

People are likely to follow someone who speaks with total self-assurance since we assume that a story told with confidence is also an accurate representation of reality. It is an effective marketing scheme, shared by New Age philosophy, to speak about a desirable future as if it already exists. Television networks advertise "the new hit of the season" before the first show is aired! Inspirational speakers, paid to elicit human potential, preach the power of purely positive thinking, and teach techniques for acting on that intention with confidence.

Of the half million rigorously controlled human studies in psychology and sociology, most ask the subject of the experiment to make a judgment of the external world as well as an estimate of his or her confidence. Perhaps the most reliable finding in all of the social sciences is that confidence is negatively correlated with accuracy. This means that the more certain one is of his judgment, the more likely he is to be wrong. All told, the correlation is close to zero though almost always negative and statistically significant. Knowing this, many states have eliminated the death penalty since juries tend to give precedence to an eyewitness account told with confidence over physical evidence presented with dispassion.

Perhaps the most reliable finding in all of the social sciences is that confidence is negatively correlated with accuracy

---

What are we to do when perceiving waves of conceit that distance us from the authority whose expertise we need? As a physician, I find it much easier to relate to patients who indicate that they do not expect omniscience but rather help in understanding themselves. The patient can give the doctor permission to be a caring, though possibly fallible, workmate. Understand, however, that those invested with authority have been selected and trained and are continually monitored by their professional societies so as to manifest authoritarian traits. For example, during medical internship we learned to leave the patient in the examination room so we could check standard references without him or her knowing. It is presumed by the medical institutions that patients will not comply with the forthcoming prescription if they discover that their doctor does not know everything in advance. For me, this relic of a secret society ended the first time that I treated a physician and we decided to work together toward the best protocol possible. Thirty minutes later we had created a plan that gave each of us a well-earned feeling of confidence.

Alexander (aka Aleister) Crowley was one of the last great British adventurers, passionately dedicated to the exploration of remote places on earth and the even more unexplored terrain of the soul. From the beginning of the twentieth century until the end of World War II, Crowley used his wealth and genius to do battle with the values of his culture, even those moral prescriptions necessary to maintain his own life and sanity.

Crowley was a prodigious writer of poetry and prose, a highly skilled rock and mountain climber, the creator of magical rites of passage, and an inveterate experimenter with drugs and sex. But whatever the project of the moment, the intention was to shake his society and, with it, his own sensibilities. To some he was a huckster (he would have appreciated the reference to Huck Finn); to others he was a prophet (a role he claimed for himself). The yellow journalism prior to the Second World War declared him "The wickedest man on Earth!" and he was proud that his personal myth was being propagated.

His friends and his enemies alike have argued that Crowley's actions were diminished by his overbearing hubris. For example, he was undoubtedly an innovative rock climber, having learned on limestone cliffs where the slightest misstep would bring you down along with a ton of rock. However, he was a liability as lead climber in Himalayan expeditions where teamwork is essential. Faced with less skilled, though somewhat arrogant, climbers, Crowley would allow them to fail, and with their loss would come the failure of the expedition.

A contemporary literary critic described Crowley's writings for the most part as second rate because his "vanity prevented him from reworking his poetry and fiction." Crowley was dedicated to understanding his every thought, word and action as a conversation with God. He reasoned, therefore, that you cannot alter so much as a comma from a divinely inspired text! This would be an example of *ratzon* rather than *hubris* if Crowley had so lost his mind to God that he could no longer see the social consequences of his acts. In fact, he relished the prospects of battle with critics he believed were unworthy to judge his work.

The Confessions of Aleister Crowley: An Autohagiography was written at the age of forty-seven, summarizing what Crowley believed was a life that had culminated in the highest spiritual realization. It should be noted that Crowley was, as always, scheming to shock the public by describing his autobiography as a hagiography (the story of a saint); at the same time he was, in all earnestness, practicing modesty by not calling it a "theography" (the story of god)! Fortunately for its readers, the style of *The Confessions* is unpretentious, and the text revealing of a man trying to break free.[2]

Crowley's life story, as is the case for most of us, interweaves the acquisition of strength and identity from one's family and culture with the need to assert one's individuality. Young Alexander and his family were devout members of the Plymouth Brethren, a Christian sect believing (a) in the literal truth of the King James Bible, (b) that priestly authority is contrary to scripture, (c) in the imminence of the Second Coming, and (d) that only those who love God and follow his Word (as elucidated by the Brethren) will enter His Kingdom. When Alexander was eleven, his father died, leaving the child to despise an unjust god, and determined to defy the divine word he had learned to accept. Inspired by images of the Apocalypse and the chastising of his exasperated mother, he began referring to himself as "The Beast."

It may be significant that, in *The Confessions,* Crowley refers to himself in the third person until his revolt against dogmatic Christianity. This suggests that even in adulthood (and supposedly as an "enlightened spirit") he was unable to accept what had happened to his father and the consequent changes in his life. A complementary explanation is that the shock of grief created a dissociative state of mind (a sense of unreality that is common when life changes so abruptly) that Crowley the biographer was able to successfully recapture.

Throughout his life, Crowley took on new names as a way of breaking with the past and announcing his aspirations. As an undergraduate student at Cambridge University he read a book that argued that famous men have names consisting of a dactyl surname followed by a trochee family name. With the echoes of Julius Caesar ringing in his imagination, he summarily changed his name from Alexander to Aleister Crowley. In subsequent years, he took on other names symbolic of his social, literary, or spiritual aspirations. For example, he became Perdurabo (meaning "I shall endure") at a time when his scholarly efforts were being harshly criticized.

Crowley was dedicated to challenging his society's "buttoned up" sense of morality. The young man had been invited to the British Museum for the ceremonial unveiling of a recently acquired Greek sculpture. ("Acquired" is here a euphemism for an arrogant society taking possession of another's creations.) Crowley was offended by the museum curator's clothing the male figure with a fig leaf, and so took the opportunity to highlight his culture's hypocrisy and "sins of restriction" by entering the ballroom wearing nothing but a fig leaf.

The older one gets, the more apparent it becomes that only an heroic, sustained, and conscious effort will allow one to set new roots. For example, Crowley disdained the King James Bible and its authoritarian prohibitions, but his writings use the same vocabulary and cadence (e.g., "Do what thou wilt shall be the whole of the Law"). Moreover, he created a new religion (Thelema, Greek for *will*) with its own bible and all the trappings of conventional Christianity. *The Book of The Law* was "revealed in epiphany" to "Perdurabo" during three days in 1904. Here is a brief excerpt.

> I am the snake that giveth Knowledge & Delight and bright glory, and stir the hearts of men with drunkenness. To worship me take wine and strange drugs whereof I will tell my

prophet, & be drunk thereof! They shall not harm ye at all. It is a lie, this folly against self. The exposure of innocence is a lie. Be strong, o man! Lust, enjoy all things of sense and rapture: fear not that any God shall deny thee for this.[3]

Since *The Book* was a divine revelation not one letter was to be altered, and the only person with the authority to interpret its meaning was Crowley.

With the mission of a prophet, Crowley eloquently set forth principles that would become New Age dogma. Namely that, with the force of will, you can do anything, making the unconscious conscious and the imagined manifest. The only obligation in life is to discover your true will. "Do what you like; not the haphazard wishes and desires of the conscious mind, but the unchangeable idea of your inner self." Supposedly, you will recognize that inner self because touching it will liberate a boundless sense of love. The New Thought, New Religious and New Age movements shared with Crowley's Thelema the belief in the magical power of words. Crowley had a first-hand understanding of the "sin of pride" and therefore required of his students a strict prohibition against using any verbal expression of self ("I," "me," "mine"), believing that such words perpetuated hubris.

Crowley took the "divine prescription" to indulge in drugs and sex quite literally, and henceforth acted on it liberally and often. In photos over the next twenty years, he ages at a remarkable rate. His indulgences aggravated his asthma and chronic bronchitis for which his physicians prescribed heroin. In order to maintain his energy and "stay up" for his poetry and sexual partners, he experimented with a variety of drugs, which aggravated further his respiratory disorders and the vicious cycle of drug use. By the time Crowley was forty-six, his addiction to heroin and cocaine made it apparent that he had misinterpreted *The Book*. In *The Fountain of Hyacinth* he reflected on the need to break the habit:

Most of my mental & moral powers were seriously affected in various ways, while I was almost wholly dependent on them for physical energy, in particular for sexual force…complicated by abnormal indulgence in alcohol. My creative life had become spasmodic & factitious…I avoided washing, dressing, shaving, as much as possible…I could not even feel alarm at obviously serious symptoms…I have erred in going too far; the worship has become forced, & fallen into fanatical frenzy which blasphemes Him. (Quoted from L. Sutin's *Do What Thou Wilt: a life of Aleister Crowley*.)[4]

The final third of Crowley's life may be seen as a series of fits and starts at revitalizing his new religion. But, he had not only lost physical and mental vitality, the world had changed. The acts of discretion so characterizing the Victorian Age had been brushed aside, the public to whom Crowley wished approbation grew easily bored with sexual innuendo, and few had energy for tantric discipline. Moreover, the world had lived through an economic depression and witnessed evil on a grand scale in the form of Nazism, leaving nothing but a voyeuristic interest in the self-styled "Beast."

It became a growing sense of frustration for Crowley that he failed to manifest his will. Few were attracted to the new dogma of Thelema, and it was painfully apparent that he could not even manage the details of his own life. He lived long enough to regret seeing his teachings turned into pornography and marketing schemes that prey on people's desire for spiritual communion or a quick, magical fix.

Crowley's reflections very much represent the human dilemma surrounding inertia and change. What appears in our youth to be striding out on our own often leads in old age to a face-to-face confrontation with our roots. Those aspects of Crowley's childhood to which he reacted so passionately launched an orbital trajectory from which he could not escape, no matter how much energy he burned. One of his last acts before heart failure was to write words of advice to his son, admonishing him to memorize as much of the Old Testament as possible.

Even if you are unable to create a new orbit for yourself, you can still, through observation and reflection, gain perspective on the ongoing story of your life. After Crowley's last visit with his teenage daughter he reflected that her uncle (who was raising her) was "annoyed & bewildered because Lion's Daughters do not grow wool! [She] is unmanageable. She despises everybody, thinks she is a genius, is stupid, inaccurate, plain, ill-tempered, etc. etc. God! But it's good to be a Lion! For the first time in my life I taste the true pleasures of immortality."

Arturo

In my first year of medical practice I was eager to demonstrate what I had learned in naturopathic school. I gave my first private patient a treatment protocol with more than twenty items to follow. The poor lady looked shocked peering at that list and, of course, I did not see her again. During that year I worked with a musician who I will call Arturo. In retrospect, his case had an undesirable outcome, not because of medical ignorance or lack of patient compliance, but because of arrogance.

Arturo was brought into my office by his wife, Gert, who released him into the chair across from me. She was a night nurse and quickly filled me in on the medical details of her husband's case. It was difficult to see that the slumped figure in a trench coat was fifty-two and of stocky build. In the space of a week, he had suffered a heart attack that required emergency room resuscitation, and two detached retinas (neither of which was related to trauma), which left the upper half of his visual field dark. He had sunk into clinical depression: not speaking, eating, or exhibiting any interest in life. She showed me a bag full of Arturo's medications intended to stabilize heart rhythm and alleviate depression.

I immediately considered how these conditions could be related. There are cases reported in the medical literature showing that abnormal muscular contraction of arteries can cause obstructions affecting blood flow to both the heart and the eyes. In turn, diminished blood flow can cause a heart attack or a detached retina. Such arterial contractions are thought to have a strong genetic component, though this could not be confirmed in Arturo's case since he had been orphaned at an early age.

Arturo deferred to his wife when asked any question. Apparently he had not had a prior history of heart or eye disorders. However, there had been signs of depression stretching back some eight years, beginning soon after his immigration to America. He had spoken "jokingly" about killing himself, apparently becoming most depressed when left alone at night.

At this point I asked if I could interview Arturo without Gert's presence, and she went into the waiting room. I began with a general inquiry "So, where do you come from?" and, with little hesitation, he commenced to tell me his story. Because he had no memory or documentation of his first years, he assumed that he was born to an unwed mother in his native Columbia, and simply abandoned.

His earliest memories were of belonging to a "pack" of street urchins, doing whatever was necessary to survive. He soon hooked up with a street musician and began learning a variety of percussion instruments. By the time he was a teenager, Arturo could count on earning his dinner by playing the marimbas for passing tourists. At the same time, he was earning the respect of townspeople and other musicians.

When he was twenty, the founding members of a rock group (an international group that is still touring and cutting CDs) came by to listen, spontaneously began jamming together, and signed him on as their percussionist. In the "golden years" that followed, Arturo lived the life of a celebrity ("wine, woman and song") and received a hero's welcome whenever he returned home.

While touring the U.S., he met and instantly fell in love with Gert. They rendezvoused a few times before discussing marriage. The lifestyle of a touring rock star was not acceptable to Gert and she posed the fateful choice: it would be either her or his music. On hearing these words, I felt a profound chill and detected an inner voice saying "No, no, don't do it!" even as the real life consequences of his decision were sitting before me.

Arturo and Gertrude married and he green-carded into the U.S. With no skills other than music, and that domain shut to him,

Arturo took a job as a school janitor, and was ever diligent in cleaning toilets. Without thinking, and in order to fill the silence, I asked, "Do you listen to music?" His eyes closed, his head down and shaking, I realized that it was too painful for him to even listen to music when forbidden to perform. At this point we were both in tears.

Can there be a more destructive form of arrogance than to ask a lover to give up that which is central to his or her identity? Spouses, often acting like parents, do this with the conviction that their "tough love" is for the loved one's benefit. But it is arrogant to ask for this and conceit to presume that we know what is best for our partners. Such an adolescent presumption is, for various reasons, doomed to failure. The task of maintaining a new persona is not a single act, like suicide, but one that requires vigilance. To accomplish this, it is necessary to either continually suppress the "old me" or sharply dissociate one's psyche into separate selves. Willfully changing one's self by staying away from that which nurtures one's "heart," sooner or later will cause psychological or physical disease, and eventually undermine any loving relationship.

For my part, I allowed my special expertise in homeopathy to distract me from my patient's social needs. It is an easy conceit to inflate the value of something to which we concentrate our energies. There is no convincing a Ph.D. candidate that his doctoral dissertation does not solve critical issues for humankind, no matter how narrowly focused the research. There is no convincing a man in love that the romance might have tragic consequences. There is no convincing a specialist in virology that a disease might not be caused by a virus. There is no convincing a child who has mastered the use of a hammer that everything he sees is not a nail. A few years ago, I saw a patient with a gum infection who had been to "the leading expert in infectious disease." The specialist had ordered a blood draw while pronouncing, to the patient's utter consternation, that it was probably HIV because he saw "at least five new cases of HIV every day." The specialist had not bothered to call back with the *negative* laboratory results, and when I spoke with him about our patient he had nothing to offer.

When I consulted with Arturo, I had recently completed my

board examination in homeopathy and published a *materia medica* of homeopathic remedies. It was, therefore, easy for me to recognize his homeopathic profile. Arturo's case, in all its detail, is a prototypic example of *Aurum*, homeopathic gold. The *Aurum* personality is depressed to the point of suicide, and dwells on such thoughts when alone and at night. There is, in their minds at least, an event after which they have never been well since. This is often the loss, in childhood, of a loving parent (in Arturo's case his being orphaned). Alternatively, they may sharply demarcate a "golden period" in their lives that was abruptly lost (Arturo's fateful choice). Besides depression, *Aurum* is a remedy used to treat eye disorders (particularly loss of vision in half of the visual field) and heart disease. The one bright spot in the heart of the *Aurum* personality is his or her love of music.

I went to the medicine cabinet and pulled out a bottle of homeopathic *Aurum* (200C potency), and gave him four pellets to suck on. Within a minute, Arturo yawned, took off his glasses and rubbed his face. He smiled and claimed that his vision had returned! With his countenance clearly improved, I called in Gert, who commented warily that she could see that "the session went well without me."

I saw them one week later and was impressed by the turn of the tide. Arturo was talkative and smiling and "trying to find ways to get music back into [his] life." In the interval, they had returned to his cardiologist and ophthalmologist, and had brought copies of their reports. The latest EKG no longer showed signs of a recent heart attack. The ophthalmologist was even more amazed because Arturo's eyesight was now restored, with only minimal signs of a retinal lesion in one eye.

As I escorted the couple out, I thought "What a great profession: find the right homeopathic pill and someone's life is changed for the better!" That Gert was looking somewhat pensive should have alerted me to trouble in paradise. The next time I heard from them was a telephone call made by Gert to my office. Arturo was insisting on playing or teaching music. Since Gert would have nothing of such a "breach of contract," she had driven him to Salt Lake City to consult with the Church Elders. From what must have been a telephone booth, I could hear in the background a snappy beat being pounded out and Gert saying "They're coming to take him away."

I only saw Arturo once more, and that only when running into the couple one afternoon. He was slumped on a bench, looking both depressed and overmedicated. Gert informed me that he was now receiving "real medicine."

My conceit was believing that a pill, however well chosen, could change someone's life. Yes, *Aurum* reawakened in Arturo his love of music and the need to reconnect with it. But, the very factors that had led to his renunciation of music and the move toward suicidal depression were still in place. I caused him to awaken a nightmarish conflict to which there was no ready resolution. In retrospect, the situation called for a therapist to work with the *couple* so as to first set the foundation for meaningful change. This would have been anything but a quick fix given the need for both party's long-term commitment to healing. However, therapy might have restored some balance of power in the couple, along with some semblance of Arturo's pride.

Contemporary homeopaths complain that their remedies don't work for as long as they used to. The blame is most often directed at today's toxic environment. But, the nineteenth and early twentieth centuries in Europe and America (the core of the industrial revolution and the classical period of homeopathy) was the most polluted time the world has known. It is significant that the mature Samuel Hahnemann offered homeopathic remedies *after* the patient had eliminated the cause of the problem and had in other ways set the groundwork for change. In cases where the cause was unknown, he asked for a "pure" lifestyle in combination with homeopathic medications that served to make the underlying cause apparent.

Part of the problem today in achieving optimal health care is that physicians are overly conceited about the relevance of their own specialty diagnoses and treatments. More time to listen to a patient's story and conduct the detective work necessary to address the cause would help, as would sufficient self-confidence and encouragement so as to reach beyond his or her acknowledged expertise. But the obstacles to achieving good health extend beyond the physician to our cultural paradigms. In particular, there is the unfortunate assumption, shared by patients and physicians, that there is, or could possibly be, an appropriate medication to fix any symptom or medical condition. Most often, the argument in the so-called "holistic" community is that the best pill is whole and natural, while pharmaceutically-oriented medicine argues for the virtues of synthetic pills that can be better standardized. The marketing world has no doubt that we live in a "pill society." Just consider the television commercial that instructs potential patients to "Ask your doctor about the purple pill."

The solution, periodically rediscovered throughout medical history, is that while medications may alleviate suffering as the body-mind complex gets its act together, and may even assist in restoring balance or helping to discover the underlying cause of the disease, only new behaviors or the move to a new environment will bring a lasting improvement in health. We may addend to this ancient prescription, from what we now know of social psychology and body-mind medicine, the ability of improved social relationships to heal.

Spiro, Antonia and Miranda

Antonia brought her fifteen-year-old daughter into my inner office, explaining as they sat down that she was worried about Miranda's health. Miranda had not had a menstrual period in over three years. She appeared lean and athletic. I asked what if anything had changed since then. Miranda answered, "Well, I play sports now; mostly soccer."

"Have you ever been significantly heavier or thinner than you are now?"

"I don't know."

Antonia added in a whisper matching her daughter's, "I think we did have a bit of a weight problem."

"Miranda, I'd bet that since you now play sports you're in better shape than when you were twelve."

"Well, yeah."

Since their gynecologist was able to rule out disease, I thought it likely that the problem had to do with a low level of body fat. I explained that estrogen is stored in fat cells and that, because of this, athletic women often do not have periods.

Antonia responded to my evaluation by standing up and declaring "Thank you, I'm sure Miranda will start eating more and getting more rest." Before letting this duo loose I told Miranda that I'd like to see her play soccer sometime, and asked them about the rest of the family. Without hesitation, Antonia described her husband, Spiro, as "a genius who always has people asking him to speak about the American Revolution. Those people don't know he can't even remember our birthdays." I asked if he was happy, and Antonia shrugged. "He stays busy. We all stay busy."

Four years later Antonia arranged for me to see Spiro in regard to his recent diagnosis of Alzheimer's disease (AD). A tall and dignified figure, he approached with both hands outstretched, asking me as an old confidant might, "So how are you today?" He had obviously developed a proactive approach to his loss of memory, but I could tell from his expression that Spiro hadn't a clue as to who I was or why he was in my office.

Antonia filled me in on the details while her husband sat nodding with a vacant smile. One week ago, Spiro had been given early retirement from the history department at Stanford University. He had been a tenured professor whose teaching and publications had earned him respect within the academic world. But, starting at about the age of sixty, he found it progressively more difficult to manage his academic responsibilities, and now, at sixty-two, he could no longer conduct a coherent lecture, nor could he reliably counsel students.

As a member of the Stanford faculty, Spiro had taken advantage of the medical school facilities. He is one of the few AD patients whose diagnosis was confirmed by brain biopsy while they were still alive. The microscopic structure of samples taken from his hippocampus and forebrain showed a significant decrease in density of nerve cell connections known as "dendrites," as well as the characteristic "tangles" and "plaques."

A sticky, cholesterol-rich plaque is found about the neurons of

AD patients. Such plaque begins in the hippocampus, a small sea-horse shaped area used to help make sense of a story or make new information permanently available. From the hippocampus, the plaque typically spreads to the forebrain (responsible for planning and creative thought) and eventually to almost all of the brain. The plaque inhibits the transmission of electrochemical messages from cell to cell and causes neurons to lose structural integrity. Neurons, like all tissue cells, have fibers running their length that give them structure. In the AD patient, the fibers become progressively tangled until they eventually strangle the life out of the cell.

The hippocampus has specialized cells that respond to estrogen and to the neurotransmitters acetylcholine and serotonin. Acetylcholine is an excitatory molecule, while serotonin helps to modulate mood and brain activity. All of these molecules are decreased in AD patients. Sometimes the low hormone and neuro-transmitter levels are caused by loss of functioning cells; other times, low levels of these chemicals contribute to the onset of AD. Either way, a vicious cycle begins in which chemical and structural deficits feed off each other.

AD patients first notice a problem with their ability to recall names or recent events. As the disease spreads, frustration gives way to lack of emotion. Anatomically, this is because the hippocampus is directly connected to the limbic system, the physical site of emotional experience. In advanced stages, there is loss of long-term memory and, sometimes, progression to total non-responsiveness. Because AD does not affect the cerebellum (at the back of the brain), there is no loss of fine motor coordination or motor memory. Consequently, patients can, for example, play a musical instrument they had learned prior to the disease, though lack the emotional expressiveness with which they had once played.

A number of pharmaceuticals have been designed to prevent plaque from forming on neurons, and we might expect them to be as successful as drugs that prevent LDL cholesterol from coating arteries. I believe it is a more profitable question to ask *why* the body produces and lays down plaque on nerve cells critical for its functioning. The general answer is that plaque formation is an adaptive response to free-radical damage. Damage can come from infections (e.g., the herpes virus), a brain concussion, minor strokes, or heavy metal toxicity (aluminum or copper). Having the APOE3 or APOE4 gene, significantly increases the risk of AD, especially in women. These genes increase peroxidation of the fatty membranes that line nerve cells, and are, therefore, a source of free-radical damage.

Signs and symptoms of AD do not develop unless there is impairment in the ability to protect and regenerate nerve tissue.

Importantly, all of the above risk factors may be present without permanent nerve damage or the symptoms of AD. Signs and symptoms of AD do not develop unless there is impairment in the ability to protect and regenerate nerve tissue. Estrogen, progesterone, melatonin, DHEAS, and nerve growth factor (NGF), all serve to prevent AD. The various hormones complement each other nicely. Estrogen promotes the production of nerve growth factor, which is essential to the regeneration of new dendrites and the excitatory molecule acetylcholine.[5] Progesterone promotes the neurotransmitters serotonin and GABA, helping us to let go of stress.[6,7] More generally, estrogen is synergistic with progesterone in preventing healthy nerve tissue from oxidizing.[8] For example, studies show that estrogen and progesterone supplementation by men or women speeds recovery from stroke or brain trauma. Injury tears tissue and dissociates its molecules, setting loose oxygen free-radicals. Progesterone prevents oxidation while estrogen acts as an antioxidant, binding with, and thereby neutralizing, the free-radicals.[9,10] Clinical supplementation with natural estrogen and progesterone has yielded some evidence for benefiting cognitive functioning in women with menopausal symptoms.

The brain neurotransmitter and antioxidant, melatonin, is essential to cleaning up free-radical fragments that accompany a bacterial or viral infection. Promoting melatonin production or supplementing with melatonin has been shown in animal and human studies to stop the progression of dementia when there is depression or a history of repeated infections.[11,12]

The hormone DHEAS is synthesized by the adrenal glands and the brain, though its production decreases dramatically with age. It prevents the peroxidation of the myelin nerve sheath, serves to elevate estrogen (and testosterone) levels, can alleviate clinical depression, and balances out the negative effects of other stress hormones. There is both animal and human evidence that the AD brain uses DHEAS at a higher rate than does the healthy brain.[13] It is particularly drawn upon, even to the point of becoming depleted, when there is depression or a high level of cortisol.

The development of AD and atherosclerosis have some features in common. For example, in both diseases either elevated homocysteine levels or a deficiency in folic acid slows the regeneration of scarred tissue, leaving the body to lay down cholesterol-rich plaque to fill the holes. Since folic acid is scarce in our diets, it is desirable to take a daily supplement.

The theory behind the science of neurology has changed profoundly over the past thirty years. In 1960 I was taught that our nervous systems are complete at the age of eleven, and that thereafter we have only to look forward to a progressive degeneration leading to dementia. (This may reflect a general medical paradigm, in that conventional wisdom of that same period also erroneously believed that the thymus gland begins to degenerate in childhood, until, by seventy, one has exhausted the body's reservoir of immune defense.) By the 1980s, it became clear that nerve dendrites continue to grow throughout life, and by 2000 there was evidence that whole neurons can regenerate.

What makes neurons grow and regenerate? The combination of balanced hormones, nerve growth factor, and exercise. With positron emission tomography or functional MRI we can see the flow of blood moving from area to area of the brain as one exercises his or her cognitive abilities. With the increased blood flow to those specific brain cells comes increased oxygen levels, improved nutrition, and elimination of toxic waste. In some ways, thinking is like pumping iron. In both, we perform an act that directs blood to a particular area of the body and in so doing preserve or expand our ability to function. In both cases, chemistry by itself has little benefit. All the calcium or magnesium we can possibly consume will not add bone without resistance exercise. Similarly, even a perfect balance of hormones and NGF will not stop AD progression without the use of your mind.

Spiro did not have some of the prominent risk factors commonly associated with AD. At this relatively young age, women are twice as likely to exhibit symptoms of AD. He has also spent his life in intellectual pursuits, which helps to keep the brain and mind functioning at a high level. It was possible that Spiro was applying his intellectual and social skills to camouflaging his deficits, much as he had on first greeting me.

But this leaves open the question of why his brain's cellular structure was being swallowed up. Even if Spiro had the APOE3 gene, it contributes little to AD in men. Antonia informed me that her husband had had no injuries to his head. This left the possibility of toxic or infectious agents. We know, for example, that the risk of dementia in general and AD in particular is doubled when one's drinking water contains aluminum (greater than 0.1mg/liter).[14] Animal experiments also show that aluminum exposure causes neurofibrillary tangles.[15] In regard to viral agents, Spiro had had a painful bout of herpes zoster (shingles) about ten years ago. The herpes virus eventually retreats from the skin into the central nervous system, and from there can quietly cause oxidative damage to the brain.

"Did you do anything that may have affected your health about two years ago, when cognitive loss first became noticeable?" At Antonia's urging, Spiro had given up cigarettes and had dieted to the point of losing forty pounds. Though these are typically considered healthy changes, they might have aggravated Spiro's AD. Nicotinic acetylcholine, an excitatory neurotransmitter that is molecularly similar to tobacco's nicotine, protects neurons from plaque.[16] In fact, tobacco smoking decreases the risk of AD (though it increases the risk of vascular dementia). Burning fat cells during a weight-loss diet can decrease estrogen levels, as had been discussed with Miranda some years earlier. It can also dump toxic residues or heavy metals that had been sequestered away in the fat cells, allowing them to resettle in the nervous system.

I recommended to Spiro and Antonia that he attempt to stay intellectually engaged since this would bring a healthy blood flow through areas of the brain that were being challenged. Since Spiro knew how to play the piano, I suggested that he be encouraged to do so. I noticed that his fidgeting hands annoyed Antonia, and so I suggested, with her nod of approval, that he take up pipe smoking. To both proposals there was a smile of recognition from Spiro.

In addition, antioxidants would be important. Vitamin E is an antioxidant for the brain that protects neurons from peroxidation. One thousand international units of vitamin E, taken with breakfast and dinner, has been shown to delay onset of advanced AD by about eight months.[17,18] Rosemary oil works in the same way as vitamin E, and has the potential to be even more effective.

Several amino acids serve to rejuvenate nerve cells. A number of well-controlled animal and human studies point to L-carnitine, showing that it can stop progression of AD in patients younger than sixty-five years of age.[19,20,21] L-carnitine works by increasing neuro-hormones, brain energy and metabolism, and the number of dendritic connections. L-proline serves to increase dendrite density and the production of L-carnitine. Glycine enhances the effectiveness of L-proline, increases acetylcholine levels in the hippocampus, and facilitates liver detoxification.[22] I recommended that Spiro take a total of 3000 mg of acetyl-carnitine, 3000 mg of glycine, and 5000 mg of L-proline each day. At this dose of L-proline, there is the added benefit that aluminum is forced out of the cells.

Which foods raise levels of these amino acids? Eggs and wheat germ are rich sources, though the highest concentrations of L-proline and L-carnitine are found in a component of colostrum known as colostrinin. In one experiment with AD patients, those taking colostrinin improved or stabilized during the following year, while those taking the placebo worsened.[23] I instructed Antonia that her husband should not eat pork, beef or MSG since these foods lower levels of the beneficial amino acids.

Spiro was already taking Ginkgo Biloba,[24] and I suggested another herb as well. Melissa (Lemon Balm), a Western herb traditionally used to stimulate the mind, is the plant with the highest concentration of nicotinic acetylcholine.[25] A recent study with healthy, young adults found that within hours of taking a standardized extract of Melissa, memory performance was significantly improved as well as an increased perception of a state of calmness.[26]

Spiro, Antonia and Miranda returned to my office four weeks later. Spiro cradled his pipe like an old pro. He said, "I just learned that you helped my daughter four years ago. Thank you, Dr. Reynolds." The false bravado was gone, and in its place was an intense look that I can only describe as "being connected." Earlier that week they had visited his neurologist who had retested Spiro's memory for a short (and uninteresting) story. Where Spiro had previously recalled only two out of eight ideas, he could now recall six. He was now able to carry on a conversation, which necessitates understanding and storing ideas long enough to think about them and construct an appropriate reply. The latest scan showed slightly improved blood flow to the hippocampus and forebrain. Spiro joked that his neurologist appeared eager to autopsy his brain but would have to wait. The best guess is that his protocol had caused his brain to dump neurotoxins. I explained that it would now be up to Spiro to revitalize his hippocampus by creating new memories.

Antonia informed me that Spiro had applied to have his university tenure reinstated. He added that he would be resuming supervision of graduate students immediately but that he would not be lecturing for at least two semesters. I asked, "I suppose this means that you'll be back on the American Revolution lecture circuit?" Spiro answered, "Not in the near future." Smiling with Antonia and Miranda, he added, "I think we've had our own revolution."

I saw Spiro and Miranda about a year later. He was between

semesters and helping his daughter and new son-in-law to move. Antonia was busy as a graduate student in mathematics. They were obviously proud that mom was the oldest person to have ventured into that field at her university. As we walked out to the parking lot Miranda made the off-hand comment, "I don't know if you've noticed, but everyone is a lot happier now."

In the course of a life there are periods when the will appears to be a chaotic and whimsical bag of desires, much as described by Heiman's assumption discussed in Chapter One. At other times, the will is experienced as the heroic effort needed to meet a challenge or the ecstasy of achieving harmony with a "higher self," as declared by Crowley. There are also times when we realize that will, as an organizing sense of where to find one's self, is always present. For both Arturo and Spiro there was a sense of will that persisted even after having lost the power to make meaningful choices. In this context, will is rarely the content of consciousness, but rather the beacon that day and night lights the external world and reflects our cognitions. It is like the sound of blood rushing through your ears, heard only in total silence; it is a diaphanous whisper reminding you of home, heard only when the rest of the mind is left in peace.

ENDNOTES

Chapter One: Inertia, Change and Choice

1. Heiman GW. *Understanding research methods and statistics: an integrated introduction for psychology.* 2nd Edition, Houghton Mifflin, 2001.
2. Milgram S. "Behavioral study of obedience." *J. Abnorm. Soc. Psychol.* 1963, 67: 371-8.
3. Bryant RA, Panesetis P. "Panic symptoms during trauma and acute stress disorder." *Behav Res Ther.* 2001, 39(8): 961-6.
4. Bly, R. *Iron John: A book about men.* Addison-Wesley, 1990.
5. Ikemi Y, Nakagawa S. "A psychosomatic study of contagious dermatitis." *Kyushu J Med Sci.* 1962, 13: 335-50.

6. Plaisance KI, Kudaravalli S, Wasserman SS, Levine MM, Mackowiak PA. "Effect of antipyretic therapy on the duration of illness in experimental influenza A, Shigella sonnei, and Rikettsia rickettsii infections." *Pharamacotherapy.* 2000, 20(12): 1417-22.

Chapter Two: I Can't Stop...

1. Ridker PM, Hennekens CH, Buring JE, Rifai N. "C-reactive protein and other markers of inflammation in the prediction of cardiovascular disease in women." *N Eng J Med* 2000, 342(12): 836-43.
2. Paterniti S, Zureik, M, Ducimetiere, P, Touboul, PJ, Feve JM, Alperovitch, A. "Sustained anxiety and 4-year progression of carotid atherosclerosis." *Arterioscler Thromb Vasc Biol* 2001, 21.
3. McCartney N. "Role of resistance training in heart disease." *Med Sci Sports Exerc* 1998, 30(10 Suppl): S396-S402.
4. Albert CM, Campos H, Stampfler MJ, Ridker PM, Manson JE, Willett WC, Ma J. "Blood levels of long-chain n-3 fatty acids and the risk of sudden death." *N Eng J Med* 2002, 346(15): 1113-8.
5. Lazarou J, Pomeranz BH, Corey PN. "Incidence of adverse drug reactions in hospitalized patients: a meta-analysis of prospective studies." *JAMA.* 1998, 279(15): 1200-5.
6. Starfield, B. "Is US health really the best in the world?" *JAMA.* 2000, 284(4): 483-485.
7. Robbins J, Hirsch C, Whitmer R, Cauley J, Harris T. "The association of bone mineral density and depression in an older population." *J Am Geriatr Soc.* 2001, 49(6): 732-6.
8. Cizza G, Ravn P, Chrousos GP, Gold PW. "Depression: a major, unrecognized risk factor for osteoporosis?" *Trends Endocrinol Metab.* 2001, 12(5): 198-203.
9. Fujita T, Ohgitani S, Nomura M. "Fall of blood ionized calcium on watching a provocative TV program and its prevention by active absorbable algal calcium (AAA CA)." *J Bone Miner Metab* 1999 17(2): 131-6.

10. Swezey RL, Swezey A, Adams J. "Isometric progressive resistive exercise for osteoporosis." *J Rheumatol* 2000, 27(5): 1260-4.

11. Winett RA, Carpinelli RN. "Potential health-Related Benefits of Resistance Training." *Prev Med* 2001, 33(5): 503-513.

12. Dimsdale JE, Herd JA. "Variability of plasma lipids in response to emotional arousal." *Pscychosom Med* 1982, 44(5): 413-30.

13. Lyness, SA. "Predictors of differences between Type A and B individuals in heart rate and blood pressure reactivity." *Psychol Bull* 1993, 114(2): 266-95.

14. Rommelspacher H, Siemanowitz B, Mannel M. "Acute and chronic actions of a dry methanolic extract of hypericum perforatum and a hyperforin-rich extract on dopaminergic and serotonergic neurons in rat nucleus accumbens." *Pharmacopsychiatry* 2001, 34 Suppl 1: S119-26.

15. Schulz V. "Clinical trials with hypericum extracts in patients with depression – results, comparisons, conclusions for therapy with antidepressant drugs." *Phytomedicine* 2002, 9(5): 468-74.

16. Woelk H. "Comparison of St. John's wort and Imipramine for treating depression: randomised controlled trial." *BMJ* 200, 321(7260): 536-9.

17. Chen S, Lin Y, Meng Q, Chen Y, Cui Z, Lu Z, Xuan W, Xie Z, Xu J, Liu C, Liu Y, Wang Y, Sun Q, Li Y, Wang S. "Comparative study on the mechanism of formation of pulse manifestations in coronary heart disease and hematopathic patients." *J Trad Chin Med* 1996, 16(2): 143-46.

18. Mckenna MC, Zevon MA, Corn B, Rounds J. "Psychosocial factors and the development of breast cancer: a meta-analysis." *Health Psychol* 1999, 18(5): 520-31.

19. Price MA, Tennant CC, Butow PN, Smith RC, Kennedy SJ, Kossoff MB, Dunn SM. "The role of psychosocial factors in the development of breast carcinoma: Part II. Life event stressors, social support, defense style, and emotional control and their interactions." *Cancer* 2001, 91(4): 686-97.

20. Medalie JH, Goldbourt U. "Angina pectoris among 10,000 men. Psychosocial and other risk factors as evidenced by a multivariate analysis of a five-year incidence study." *Am J Med* 1976, 60(6): 910-21.
21. Itkowitz NI, Kerns RD, Otis JD. "Support and coronary heart disease: the importance of significant other responses." *J Behav Med* 2003, 26(1): 19-30.
22. King KB, Reis HT, Porter LA, Norsen LH. "Social support and long-term recovery from coronary artery surgery: effects on patients and spouses." *Health Psychol* 1993, 12(1): 56-63.
23. Pennebaker JW, Susman JR. "Disclosure of traumas and psycho-somatic processes." *Soc Sci Med* 1988, 26(3): 327-32.
24. Petrie KJ, Booth RJ, Pennebaker JW. "The immunological effects of thought suppression." *J Pers Soc Psychol* 1998, 75(5): 1264-72.
25. Sadzuka Y, Sugiyama T, Hirota S. "Modulation of cancer Chemotherapy by green tea." *Clin Cancer Res* 1998, 4: 153-6.
26. Matsunaga H, Katano M, Saita T, Yamamoto H, Mori M. "Potent-iation of cytotoxicity of mitomycin C by a polyacetylenic alcohol, panaxytiol." *Cancer Chemother Pharmacol* 1994, 33(4): 291-7.
27. Gogos CA, Ginopoulos P, Salsa B, Apostolidou E, Zoumbos NC, Kalfarentzos, F. "Dietary omega-3 polyunsaturated fatty acids plus vitamin E restore immunodeficiency and prolong survival for severely ill patients with generalized malignancy: a random-ized control trial." *Cancer* 1998, 82(2): 395-402.

Chapter Three: Never Well Since...

1. Lange U, Jung O, Teichmann J, Neek G. "Relationship between disease activity and serum levels of vitamin D metabolites and parathyroid hormone in ankylosing spondylitis." *Osteoporos* Int. 2001, 12(12): 1031-5.
2. Falkenback A, Tripathi R, Sedlmeyer A, Staudinger M, Herold M. "Serum 25-hydroxyvitamin D and parathyroid hormone in patients with ankylosing spondylitis before and after a three-week rehabilitation treatment at high altitude during winter and spring." *Wien Klin Wochenschr.* 2001, 113(9): 328-32.

3. Cousins, N. *Anatomy of an illness as perceived by the patient.* Norton & Co., 1979.
4. McKenna MC, Zevon MA, Corn B, Rounds J. Psychosocial factors and the development of breast cancer: a meta-analysis." *Health Psychol.* 1999, 18(5): 520-31.
5. Deschamps FJ, Turpin JC. "Methyl bromide intoxication during grain store fumigation." *Occup Med* (Lond). 1996, 46(1): 89-90.
6. Bensky D, Gamble A. *Chinese herbal medicine: materia medica.* Eastland Press, 1993.
7. Iwata M, Nakano H, Matsuura Y, Nagasaka M, Misawa M, Mizuta S, Ito I, Saito T, Ito T, Hokama M, Kamiya M, Hobara R, Watanabe M, Takahama K. "Intestinal permeability in Crohn's disease and effects of elemental dietary therapy." *Nippon Shokakibyo Gakkai Zasshi.* 2001, 98(6): 636-43.

Chapter Four: Relics and Fossils

1. Hoyert DL, Arias E, Smith BL, Murphy SL, Kochanek KD. "Deaths: final data for 1999." *CDC: National Vital Statistics Reports.* 2001, 49(9).
2. Spiegel D, Bloom JR, Kraemer HC, Gottheil E. "Effect of psychosocial treatment on survival of patients with metastatic breast cancer." *Lancet.* 1989, 2(8668): 888-91.
3. Stanton AL, Danoff-Burg S, Sworowski LA, Collins CA, Branstetter AD, Rodriguez-Hanley A, Kirk SB, Austefeld JL. "Randomized, controlled trial of written emotional expression and benefit finding in breast cancer patients." *J Clin Oncol.* 2002, 20(20): 4160-8.
4. Petrie KJ, Booth RJ, Pennebaker JW. "The immunological effects of thought suppression." *J Pers Soc Psychol.* 1998, 75(5): 1264-72.
5. El-Metwally TH, Adrian TE. "Optimization of treatment conditions for studying of anticancer effects of retinoids using pancreatic adenocarcinoma as a model." *Biochem Ciophys Res Commun.* 1999, 257(2): 596-603.
6. Jung, CG. *Memories, dreams, reflections.* Pantheon Books, 1973.
7. Verma V. *Ayurveda: a way of life.* Samuel Weiser, 1995.

Chapter Five: Ghosts, Gods, and Haunting Refrains

1. Jaynes J. *The origins of consciousness in the breakdown of the bicameral mind.* Houghton Mifflin, 1982.
2. Luther M., *The bondage of the will.* Baker Book House, 1999.
3. Schopenhaur A. *The world as will and idea.* Truber & Co., 1983.
4. Overbye D. *Einstein in love: a scientific romance.* Penguin Group, 2000.
5. Renn J, Schulmann R (eds.). *Albert Einstein/Mileva Maric — the love letters.* Princeton University Press, 1992.
6. Renn J, Schulmann R (eds.), ibid.
7. Lutgendorf SK, Kreder KJ, Rothrock NE, Ratliff TL, Zimmerman B. "Stress and symptomatology in patients with interstitial cystitis: a laboratory stress model." *J Urol.* 2000, 164(4): 1265-9.
8. Huxley RR. "Nausea and vomiting in early pregnancy: its role in placenta development." *Obstet Gynecol.* 2000, 95(5): 779-82.
9. Flaxman SM, Sherman PW. "Morning Sickness: a mechanism for protecting mother and embryo." *Q Rev Biol.* 2000, 75(2): 113-48.
10. Brett M, Baxendale S. "Motherhood and memory: a review." 2001, 26: 339-362.

Chapter Six: Perfection

1. Wittenberg KJ, Norcross JC. "Practitioner perfectionism: relationship to ambiguity tolerance and work satisfaction." *J Clin Psychol.* 2001, 57(12): 1543-50.
2. Cuban, L. *How teachers taught: Constancy and change in American classrooms, 1890-1990.* 2nd edition, 1993. Teachers College Press.
3. Riefenstahl L. *Leni Riefenstahl: a memoir.* St. Martin's Press, 1992.
4. Gogos CA, Ginopoulos P, Salsa B, Apostolidou E, Zoumbos NC, Kalfarentzos F. "Dietary omega-3 polyunsaturated fatty acids plus vitamin E restore immunodeficiency and prolong survival for severely ill patients with generalized malignancy: a randomized control trial." *Cancer.* 1998, 82(2): 395-402.

5. Carrillo-Vico A, Garcia-Maurino S, Calvo JR, Guerrero JM. "Melatonin counteracts the inhibitory effect of PGE2 on IL-2 production in human lymphocytes via its mt1 membrane receptor." *FASEB J.* 2003, 17(6): 755-7.

6. Mayo JC, Tan DX Sainz RM, Natarajan M, Lopez-Burillo S, Reiter RJ. "Protection against oxidative protein damage induced by metal-catalyzed reaction or alkylperoxyl radicals: comparative effects of melatonin and other antioxidants." *Biochim Biophys Acta.* 2003, 1620(1-3): 139-50.

7. Kojima T, Mochizuki C, Mitaka T, Mochizuki Y. "Effects of melatonin on proliferation, oxidative stress and Cx32 gap junction protein expression in primary cultures of adult rat hepatocytes." *Cell Stuct Funct.* 1977, 22(3): 347-56.

8. Sauer LA, Dauchy RT, Black DE. "Polyunsaturated fatty acids, melatonin, and cancer prevention." *Biochem Pharmacol.* 2001, 61(12): 1455-62.

9. Maestroni GJ. "Therapeutic potential of melatonin in immunodeficiency states, viral diseases, and cancer." *Adv Exp Med Biol.* 1999, 467: 217-26.

10. Kelder, P. *Ancient Secrets of the Fountain of Youth.* Doubleday, 1999.

Chapter Seven: Hubris

1. *Herodotus: the histories: Xerxes at the Hellespont, in reading about the world*, v. 1. Brians P, Gallwey M, Hughes D, Hussain A, Law R, Myers M, Neville M, Schlesinger R, Spitzer A, Swan S (eds.). Third edition, Harcourt Brace Custom Publishing,1999.

2. Symonds J, Grant K (eds.). *The confessions of Aleister Crowley: an autohagiography.* Hill & Wang, 1970.

3. Crowley A. *The book of the law, in the equinox of the gods.* O.T.O., 1936.

4. Sutin L. *Do what thou wilt: a life of Aleister Crowley.* St. Martin's Griffin, 2000.

5. Simpkins JW, Green PS, Gridley KE, Singh M, de Fiebre NC, Rajakumar G. "Role of estrogen replacement therapy in memory enhancement and the prevention of neuronal loss associated with Alzheimer's disease." *Am J Med.* 1977, 103(3A): 19S-25S.

6. Bethea CL, Lu NZ, Gundlah C, Streicher JM. "Diverse actions of ovarian steroids in the serotonin neural system." *Front Neuroendocrinol.* 2002, 23(1): 41-100.

7. Rupprecht R. "Neuroactive steroids: mechanisms of action and neuropsychopharmacological properties." *Psychoneuroendocrinology.* 2003, 28(2): 139-68.

8. Nilsen J, Brinton RD. "Impact of progestins on estrogen-induced neuroprotection: synergy by progesterone and 19-norprogesterone and antagonism by medroxyprogesterone acetate." *Endocrinology.* 2002, 143(1): 205-12.

9. Roof RL, Hall ED. "Gender differences in acute CNS trauma and stroke: neuroprotective effects of estrogen and progesterone." *J Neurotrauma.* 2000, 17(5): 367-88.

10. Stein DG, Hoffman SW. "Estrogen and progesterone as neuroprotective agents in the treatment of acute brain injuries." *Pediatr Rehabil.* 2003, 6(1): 13-22.

11. Jean-Louis G, von Gizycki H, Zizi F. "Melatonin effects on sleep, mood, and cognition in elderly with mild cognitive impairment." *J Pineal Res.* 1998, 25(3): 177-83.

12. Brusco LI, Marques M, Cardinali DP. "Monozygotic twins with Alzheimer's disease treated with melatonin: Case report." *J Pineal Res.* 1998, 25(4): 260-3.

13. Bastianetto S, Ramassamy C, Poirier J, Quirion R. "Dehydroepiandrosterone (DHEA) protects hippocampal cells from oxidative stress-induced damage." *Brain Res Mol Brain Res.* 1999, 66(1-2): 35-41.

14. Rondeau V, Commenges D, Jacqmin-Gadda H, Dartigues JF. *Am J Epidemiol.* 2000, 152(1): 59-66.

15. El-Rahman SS. "Neuropathology of aluminum toxicity in rats (glutamate and GABA impairment)." *Pharmacol Res.* 2003, 47(3): 189-94.

16. Maelicke A. "Allosteric modulation of nicotinic receptors as a treatment strategy for Alzheimer's disease." *Dement Geriatr Cogn Disord.* 2000, 11 Suppl, 1:11-8.

17. Sano M, Ernesto C, Thomas RG, Klauber MR, Schafer K, Grundman M, Woodbury P, Growdon J, Cotman CW, Pfeiffer E, Schneider LS, Thal LJ. "A controlled trial of selegiline, alpha-tocopherol, or both as treatment for Alzheimer's disease." *The Alzheimer's Disease Cooperative Study.* N Engl J Med. 1997, 336(17): 1216-22.

18. Behl C. "Vitamin E protects neurons against oxidative cell death in vitro more effectively than 17-beta estradiol and induces the activity of the transcription factor NF-kappaB." *J Neral Transm.* 2000, 107(4): 393-407.

19. Thal LJ, Cara A, Clarke WR Ferris SH, Friedland RP, Petersen RC, Pettegrew JW, Pfeiffer E, Rasking MA, Sano M, Tuszynski MH, Woolson RF. "A 1-year multicenter placebo-controlled study of acetyl-L-carnitive in patients with Alzheimer's disease." *Neurology.* 1996, 47(3): 705-11.

20. Brooks JO 3rd, Yesavage JA, Carta A, Bravi D. "Acetyl L-carnitine slows decline in younger patients with Alzheimer's disease: a reanalysis of a double-blind, placebo-controlled study using the trilinear approach." *Int Psychogeriatr.* 1998, 10(2): 193-203.

21. Pettegrew JW, Levine J, McClure RJ. "Acetyl-L-carnitine physical-chemical, metabolic, and therapeutic properties: relevance for its mode of action in Alzheimer's disease and geriatric depression." *Mol Psychiatry.* 2000, 5(6): 616-32.

22. Baxter MG, Lanthorn TH, Frick KM, Golski S, Wan RQ, Olton DS. "D-cycloserine, a novel cognitive enhancer, improves spatial memory in ages rates." *Neurobiol Aging.* 1994, 15(2): 207-13.

23. Leszek J, Inglot AD, Janusz M, Lisowski J, Krukowska K, Georgiades JA. "Colostrinin: a proline-rich polypeptide (PRP) complex isolated from ovine colostrum for treatment of Alzheimer's disease. A double-blind, placebo-controlled study." *Arch Immunol Ther Exp (Warsz).* 1999, 47(6): 377-85.

24. Wettstein A. "Cholinesterase inhibitors and Gingko extracts—are they comparable in the treatment of dementia? Comparison of published placebo-controlled efficacy studies of at least six month's duration." *Phytomedicine.* 2000, 6(6): 393-401.
25. Wake G, Court J, Pickering A, Lewis R, Wilkins R, Perry E. "CNS acetylcholine receptor activity in European medicinal plants traditionally used to improve failing memory." *J Ethnopharmacol.* 2000, 69(2): 105-14.
26. Kennedy DO, Wake G, Savelev S, Tildesley NT, Perry EK, Wesnes KA, Scholey AB. "Modulation of mood and cognitive performance following acute administration of single doses of Melissa Officinalis (Lemon Balm) with human CNS nicotinic and muscarinic receptor-binding properties." *Neuropsychopharmacology.* 2003, Oct. 28(10): 1871-81.

INDEX

B

behaviorism: 2
Bly, Robert: 8
Bombyx processiana (homeopathic): 84
breathing exercises: *See Pranayama*
Buddha: 120

C

Calcarea carbonica (homeopathic): 140-141
cancer
    anti-cancer diet: 100, 153-155
    basic therapy: 98-102, 153-157
    breast: 62, 96-103, 125
    immune system and: 55-57
    ovarian: 152-156
    pancreatic: 57-58
    patient-doctor interaction and: 171
    perfectionism and: 157-158, 160-161
    risk factors: 26, 50-52
    See also Type C personality
Celeste: 111-116
Charaka: 12-13
cholesterol: 24, 25-28, 30, 42, 127, 189
Charcot, Jean: 9
cheilitis: 161-163, 166-169
Chronic Fatigue Syndrome (CFS): 72-81
cognitive-behavioral psychology: 2-3, 29, 128

conditioning
    Pavlovian: 2, 128
    Skinnerian: 12, 128
confidence: 142, 175-177, 187
consciousness: 2, 3, 17, 75, 83, 84, 111, 161, 196
corticosteroids: *see* steroids
Cousins, Norman: 59-62
Crohn's disease (CD): 85, 87-89
Crowley, Aleister: 178-183
Crystel: 124-133
cystitis
    honeymoon: 74-75
    interstitial: 126-127, 129

D

David: 82-84
depression: 7, 20, 35, 37, 41, 43, 45, 56, 74, 94-95, 124, 162, 184, 192
    anxious: 6, 21, 39, 42, 45, 89, 98, 107, 135
Descartes, Rene: 2-3
Determinism: 3-4
detoxification: 66-67, 72, 106-107, 134
Doctor Shiva: 71-72
Dosha: 12
    See also, Kapha, Pitta, Vata

E

Einstein, Albert: 120-124, 141
Einstein-Maric, Mileva: 120-124
"Elemental Diet": 89
estrogen: 13, 25, 28, 95, 152-153, 189, 191-192

evidence-based medicine: 95-96

F
fibromyalgia: 80-81
Frances: 63-71
Frank: 139-143
Freud, Sigmund: 9, 19-21, 29

G
GABA: 43, 45, 94-95, 136, 190-191
Gilgamesh: 173-174
Glycemic Index: 31-33

H
Hahnemann, Samuel: 82, 187
health
    challenges to: 19, 21, 29, 35,
        97-98, 101, 170-171, 174-
        175, 187-188
    characteristics of: 9, 22-23, 26,
        97-98, 151-152
    promoting of: 8, 13, 31, 53,
        61, 63, 108, 114, 158, 161,
        167, 174-175
Hemingway: Ernest: 93-95
Hippocrates: 12-13, 15, 22, 82
Hitler, Adolf: 149
homeopathic portraits: *See specific*
   remedies
homeopathy: 22, 29, 31, 82-84,
   116-117, 128, 139, 187
hubris: 172-176
hypnosis: 8, 9, 48-50, 71, 131-132
hypotension, orthostatic (postural): 74

I
imbalances: 22-24, 47, 63
inertia: 7, 41,93, 108, 140, 173,
   182
influence paradigm: 4-6, 85, 93,
   63
influenza: 15
insomnia: 10-11, 24, 28, 37

K
Jackie: 72-82
Jaynes, Julian: 119
Jerazad: 96-103
Jung, Carl: 105

K
Kapha: 22, 48, 168

L
leaky gut: 80, 139
Lila: 105-111
Lilith: 34-41
love, as health-promoting: 52-53,
   56-58, 62, 81, 101-103, 106,
   109, 111, 124-125, 133, 145,
   185
Louis: 50-58
Luther, Martin: 119
Lycopodium (homeopathic): 142-
   143

M
Maria: 133-138
Marsha: 103-104
melatonin: 37-38, 67, 98, 99,
   155-157, 191, 192

ABOUT THE AUTHOR

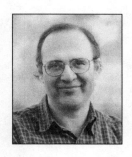

Robert Reynolds, Ph.D., N.D.

Since 1976, Dr. Reynolds has been a professor of psychology at prestigious universities in the U.S. and abroad, including Yeshiva University (NYC), Antioch University (Southern California), Fordham (NYC), and Rutgers (New Jersey). He is trained and licensed as a Naturopathic Physician, and certified in Homeopathy. Dr. Reynolds is also an International Chess Master.

He is currently in private practice in Santa Barbara and Santa Ynez, California, and teaches Health Sciences at Santa Barbara City College. He is a research consultant for "Healing Opportunities," a non-profit organization promoting research and education in complementary medicine. Dr. Reynolds is dedicated to integrating Western and Eastern medical knowledge and empowering people to choose the complement of therapies most consistent with personal philosophy and life situations.

Contact Information: Dr. Reynolds can be reached c/o: Hohm Press, PO Box 31, Prescott, Arizona, 86302.

Tarique: 161-169
Telemachus [or Telly]: 85-91
Tong-Len: 159-160
transference, psychodynamic: 128
Type A personality: 42-43, 53
Type C personality: 52-53, 81

U
ulcers: 10-11

V
Vata: 22, 48, 75, 168
vicious cycle: 11-12
vitamin D: 30, 36, 61, 88, 98,
   99, 112

W
weight loss, diet for: 33, 34, 75,
   85, 127, 194

Wilber, Ken: 3
will: 2-5, 6, 61-62, 93, 108-109,
   119-120, 133, 145, 159, 181-
   183, 196
   free: 4-5, 119-120
   God's: 119, 120, 172
   Luther's disdain for: 119
   relinquishing one's: 119, 120,
      133
   Schopenhauer's view of: 119-
      120
willful: 157, 172-174

X
Xerxes: 172-173